DATE DUE		

—Diseases and People—

MEASLES AND RUBELLA

Alvin, Virginia, and Robert Silverstein

Enslow Publishers, Inc.

40 Industrial Road   PO Box 38
Box 398   Aldershot
Berkeley Heights, NJ 07922   Hants GU12 6BP
USA   UK

http://www.enslow.com

Library of Congress Cataloging-in-Publication Data

Silverstein, Alvin.
    Measles and rubella / Alvin, Virginia, and Robert Silverstein.
       p. cm. — (Diseases and people)
    Includes bibliographical references and index.
    ISBN 0-89490-714-X
      1. Measles—Juvenile literature. 2. Rubella—Juvenile literature. I. Silverstein,
Virginia B. II. Silverstein, Robert A. III. Title. IV. Series.
RC168.M4S55 1997
616.9'15—DC21   97-3785
                                                    CIP
                                                    AC

Printed in the United States of America

10 9 8 7 6 5 4

Illustration Credits: Centers for Disease Control and Prevention, pp. 30, 78, 82,
85, 87; © 1996 Norm Rockwell, distributed by King Features Syndicate, p. 64;
Courtesy of National Library of Medicine, pp. 17, 89, 100; National Institute of
Health Photo, Courtesy of National Library of Medicine, p. 91; Portrait by Maria
Beale, Courtesy of National Library of Medicine, p. 20; "Recognize the Disease"
poster, World Health Organization, p. 35; Siena College, p. 9; WHO photo by D.
Henrioud, Courtesy of National Library of Medicine, p. 56; World Health
Organization, pp. 41, 47, 50, 55, 61, 73.

Cover Illustration: Centers for Disease Control and Prevention.

Contents

Acknowledgments

The authors would like to thank Dr. Maurice R. Hilleman, Director of Merck Institute for Therapeutic Research and Dr. Ted W. Grace, Director of Student Health Services at Ohio State University for their careful reading of the manuscript and their many helpful comments and suggestions. Their generous sharing of their expertise and their encouragement were greatly appreciated.

MEASLES

What is it? A highly contagious disease caused by a morbillivirus. Also called rubeola.

Who gets it? Mainly children, but people of any age who are not immune to the virus can catch it. In the United States today it occurs mainly in preschool children who have not been vaccinated and in schoolchildren or young adults whose immunization was not effective.

How do you get it? By breathing in moisture droplets contaminated with discharges from the nose or throat of an infected person or by touching contaminated surfaces, then touching the eyes, nose, or mouth.

What are the symptoms? Cold- or flulike symptoms beginning about ten days after exposure; fever, runny nose, cough, red eyes, and tiredness. Several days later a blotchy red rash appears on the face and spreads to the rest of the body. Complications include ear infections and pneumonia. About one in one thousand infected people develops brain inflammation (encephalitis), which may lead to mental retardation, neurological problems, behavioral disorders, or death. Symptoms tend to be more severe in teenagers and adults than in children.

How is it treated? Bed rest, fluids, acetaminophen for headache and fever, and dim lighting if the eyes are sensitive to light.

How can it be prevented? Two injections of a weakened live-virus vaccine, usually given at twelve to fifteen months of age and before entering school, provide immunity against measles in most people. (In developing countries the first shot of vaccine may be given at six to twelve months.)

RUBELLA

What is it? A contagious disease caused by a rubivirus. Also called German measles, it is less serious than measles (rubeola) except to a developing fetus; most dangerous in the first three months of pregnancy.

Who gets it? Mainly children, but people of any age who are not immune to the virus can catch it. Pregnant women can transmit the virus through the placenta to the developing fetus.

How do you get it? By breathing in moisture droplets contaminated with respiratory discharges from an infected person or by touching contaminated surfaces, then touching the eyes, nose, or mouth.

What are the symptoms? A mild rash that appears twelve to twenty-four days after exposure; headache, body aches, eye inflammation, low fever, and swollen glands may appear a week before the rash, especially in young adults. Adult women may develop arthritis lasting for several months. Children born to a woman who had rubella during the first seven months of pregnancy may suffer from congenital rubella syndrome, which may include heart defects, deafness, cataracts, glaucoma, mental retardation, slow growth, and bone disease.

How is it treated? Bed rest if needed; acetaminophen or other nonaspirin medication for pain and fever.

How can it be prevented? Immunization with rubella vaccine (usually combined with measles and mumps vaccines—MMR—for routine vaccination in childhood, or specially given to adolescent females).

1

A New Rash of Measles

At Siena College in upstate New York, the spring 1989 semester was unforgettable. Early in February, a student brought a case of measles back from a vacation in Puerto Rico. Quickly other students fell ill. A check of student health records revealed that hardly any of the 2,700 students were protected against this highly contagious disease. The college health service organized an emergency inoculation program, and within a week about twenty-nine hundred students and staff members had received measles shots.

Meanwhile, officials tried to keep the outbreak from spreading. It was not enough just to isolate the students who already had measles; others who had been exposed could also pass the germs along for a week or more before they knew they were ill. Students were urged to stay on campus, to keep from spreading the disease to people in the nearby town and in their home communities. Concerts and other public programs were cancelled. But what about the basketball season? The Siena Saints were in first place in their conference, with twenty-three straight wins at home, played before standing-room-only crowds. But crowds could spread measles germs. So the Siena team finished their season without spectators. Live television coverage allowed fans to follow the games as the team went into the NCAA play-offs.

In the month that measles laid siege to the Siena campus, twenty-six students came down with measles, along with nine people in the surrounding community and a player on an opposing basketball team. The little college made national headlines. Students printed and sold T-shirts with slogans like "Do shots—avoid the spots," and the Siena outbreak was used as a $400 clue on the TV game show, *Jeopardy*.[1]

In 1989 doctors all across the country were starting to see patients with a strange rash. Many doctors had never seen cases like these before. Between 1989 and 1991, fifty-five thousand cases of this disease were reported in the United States. It caused thousands of children and young adults to be hospitalized, and 132 died.[2] This was not a strange new disease. It was measles, once one of the most common childhood illnesses and still one of the leading causes of death of children in developing countries. Each year measles is responsible for the death of more than one million children. Or, as Dr. Robert Daum, a pediatrics professor at the University of Chicago, puts it: "Every 15 minutes, a child somewhere in the world dies because of measles."[3]

Before the 1960s, measles was so common that almost everyone caught it during the childhood years. Each year there were about half a million reported cases in the United States, and in some years nearly twice that many! Then, in the early 1960s, a vaccine was developed, and within a few years doctors saw a dramatic change. The vaccine was so successful that health officials believed the disease could be wiped out in the United States.

By 1983 the number of new cases had plunged to less than fifteen hundred—a small fraction of the usual totals twenty years before. That is why health officials and the general

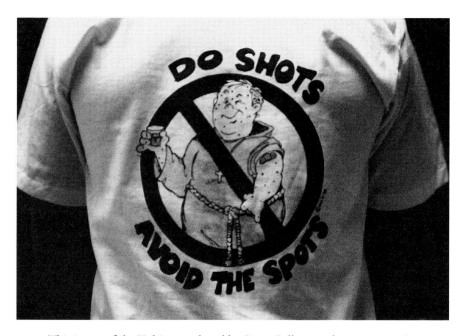

This is one of the T-shirts produced by Siena College students as souvenirs of the 1989 measles outbreak.

public were caught completely off-guard when the epidemic broke out in 1989. What had gone wrong? Why was measles making a comeback when it seemed that medicine had nearly defeated it?

The main answer to these questions is that "the U.S. has been less successful than other countries in getting the entire population immunized," as Dr. Lorry Rubin points out.[4] Dr. Rubin is the chief of infectious diseases at Schneider Children's Hospital of Long Island Jewish Medical Center in New Hyde Park, New York. But there are really two reasons for this lack of success, which is why the recent outbreaks of measles seem to be striking two main groups of victims.

In the 1989 to 1991 epidemic, many of the major outbreaks were occurring among inner-city minority children under the age of five who had never received measles vaccinations. According to the Centers for Disease Control (CDC) surveys, in many areas where outbreaks occurred, only 50 percent of two-year-olds were vaccinated.[5] "People became complacent and less vaccine was used," Dr. Donald Poretz of the National Foundation for Infectious Diseases noted in a *New York Times* interview.[6]

The other group affected by the new outbreaks included mostly college students, many of whom *had* received vaccinations as infants. It appeared that, in some cases, a single dose of the vaccine did not provide as permanent a protection as health officials had thought.

An all-out effort was launched to stop the epidemic. Health officials quickly set up emergency vaccination programs in areas hardest hit by the outbreaks, to vaccinate young children who had not received immunizations. In most states, school-age children and college students were already required to have proof of vaccination against childhood diseases such as measles. But many had received only a single measles vaccination as infants. Government health officials revised their recommendations for measles vaccinations, indicating that children should receive two vaccinations to ensure longer-lasting protection. Special clinics were set up to vaccinate children and young adults in the schools and college campuses where outbreaks had occurred.

In 1985 only 65 percent of the nation's two-year-olds had been vaccinated, but by 1991 this number had increased to 83 percent.[7] The renewed concern for immunizing children against measles quickly paid off. By the mid-1990s the number of measles cases had plunged again, to a new all-time low. Is the battle over? Health experts emphasize that fighting preventable diseases is an ongoing battle. To stay on top, the general public has to remain aware of the importance of immunization for controlling diseases. "Measles will find those who are not immunized," says Dr. Richard Duma of the National Foundation for Infectious Diseases.[8]

2

Measles and History

In the Old Testament there are many references to plagues and pestilence—periodic outbreaks of diseases that killed thousands of people. Bible scholars have traditionally assumed that "plague" referred mainly to bubonic plague, a deadly bacterial disease carried and spread by rats and fleas. Some of the biblical references to sickness pertain to leprosy, a disease that has long been feared not only because it kills but also because it can produce horrible deformities. But experts point out that the epidemics mentioned in the Bible could have been caused by any of the common infections that have troubled humanity, such as measles, smallpox, influenza, typhoid, and dysentery—all of which can cause deadly epidemics.[1]

Where Did Measles Come From?

The virus that causes measles is rather similar to the viruses that cause canine distemper in dogs and a disease called rinderpest in cattle, pigs, and hogs. Scientists believe that an ancient form of one of these viruses may have undergone mutations, or changes, that made it capable of infecting humans.[2]

Although measles is one of the world's most common diseases today, medical experts believe that it could not have become widely established until about 2,500 B.C. Unlike a disease such as bubonic plague, which bounces back and forth between infected rats and humans and is carried by fleas, measles occurs only in people. It is spread by contact between one person and another. Until the ancient Sumerian cities were built in the Middle East, there simply were not enough people living close together for a disease like measles to get a strong foothold. Among people living in small, scattered groups, a measles outbreak would tend to fade away quickly as soon as everyone who could catch it became ill. Then there would be no one else to carry on the chain of infection. Scientists have calculated that a population of about three hundred thousand to four hundred thousand people is the minimum needed for a disease like measles to become established. Once that minimum number was reached, a number of infections became common among different civilized communities in ancient Eurasia.[3]

Some diseases become so common that almost everyone gets them rather early in life. These are often called childhood diseases. Although some people die from these diseases, usually they pass without any long-lasting effects. The common childhood diseases are caused by viruses; they can be spread only by people who are actively infected, although they may have no outward signs of illness. There is a reason why such diseases tend to be relatively mild. Disease-causing viruses typically infect only certain living things (their hosts). If a virus that infects humans rapidly killed all of the people who were infected with it, soon the virus would be wiped out, too—it would have no more potential hosts to infect. So the viruses that are common today are actually very well adapted parasites—they have evolved over thousands of years to be able to infect their hosts without killing too many of them.

Diseases and Immunity

Many diseases begin in small, primitive communities, where they cause only occasional problems. These same diseases may produce epidemics when they are carried to more crowded areas. This is what has happened recently with AIDS. But for other diseases the opposite is true. Throughout history, when diseases that arose in populated areas were accidentally brought to less developed areas by explorers, missionaries, or traders, the diseases have been devastating.

After people recover from an acute infection, they are usually immune to being infected by the same kind of germ again. As a disease establishes itself in a community, the community as a whole develops a partial resistance to the disease—not enough to prevent it from occurring, but enough to make the illness less severe when a person is infected. A woman who has survived the disease can transmit protective antibodies to her unborn child and then, for a few months after birth, through her milk to the nursing baby. But in populations that have never been exposed to a particular disease germ, the first experience with it can be devastating. In these populations the disease is no longer just a childhood illness but can strike all ages because no one is immune to it.

The Beginnings of Measles

Piecing together scattered ancient writings, medical historian William McNeill put together clues as to how and when common diseases such as measles arose. McNeill concludes that the ancestors of modern childhood diseases were familiar to ancient Middle Eastern populations well before 500 B.C. The diseases played a role in reducing the population from time to time, and sometimes they helped to change the course of wars. But the diseases did not significantly reduce the general population between the ninth and fifth centuries B.C., when the biblical writers put the Old Testament into its current form.

It was during this period, in the densely populated regions of the Middle East, that some of the common modern childhood diseases had become established. Epidemics periodically occurred in the outlying regions when unusual conditions arose, such as battles where large groups of people gathered in very close quarters. The sudden outbreaks were devastating enough to attract the attention of the priests and scribes who wrote the biblical texts of the ancient world.[4]

By 500 B.C., however, common diseases such as measles had not yet spread to the Mediterranean region, where the Greek culture was thriving. Hippocrates, the father of Greek medicine, who lived from 460 to 377 B.C., described case histories of many different diseases. Modern medical experts recognize some of his descriptions as mumps, malaria, diphtheria, tuberculosis, and influenza. However, measles was not among the numerous diseases Hippocrates described.[5]

By the end of the ninth century A.D., the Persian physician Abu Bakr Muhammad ibn Zakariyā, known as al-Rhazes of Baghdad, was familiar with epidemic diseases involving skin rashes. In fact, measles was so common that al-Rhazes did not realize it was an infectious disease. He thought it was a normal part of childhood, like losing baby teeth.[6] Al-Rhazes's descriptions are the earliest written record of measles that modern historians have found, but he referred to writings from several centuries before.[7] Measles was common among Mediterranean populations in the second to third centuries A.D., and major epidemics occurred in the Roman Empire at this time.[8] Measles is thought to have arrived in China, another center of human civilization in the ancient world, in the fourth century A.D. Soon major epidemics were occurring there, too.[9]

Measles in Europe

During the Middle Ages, both measles and smallpox gradually spread throughout Europe. By the sixteenth century, they had

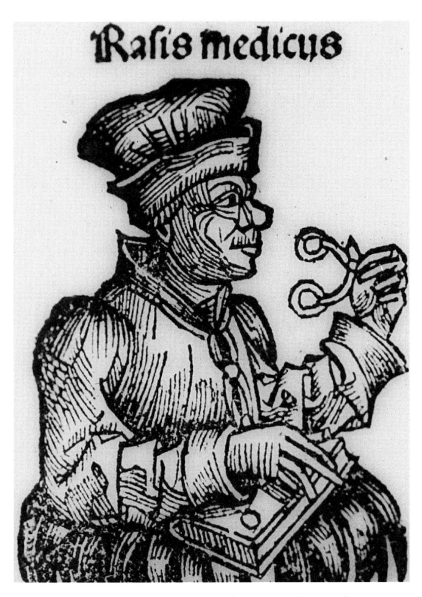

Abu Bakr Muhammad ibn Zakariyā, the Persian physician known as al-Rhazes of Baghdad, described measles back in the ninth century.

established themselves as common childhood diseases all across the European continent.[10] Although al-Rhazes had written of measles and smallpox as two separate diseases, they were often confused with each other and with other diseases characterized by rashes until the seventeenth century. Death reports by parish clerks in London in 1629 had separate listings for measles and smallpox.[11] William Shakespeare referred to measles and its transmission from person to person in his drama *Coriolanus*.[12] A British physician named Thomas Sydenham observed symptoms of an epidemic that spread throughout London around 1670 and published a medical description of measles.[13]

THE LANGUAGE OF MEASLES

The Persian physician al-Rhazes called measles *hasbah*, meaning "eruption," or "rash." He distinguished between measles and smallpox, but he thought that they had the same cause. The word "measles" first appeared in the English language in the fourteenth century. It came from the word "miser" (misery), which was the way writers referred to the terrible condition of lepers.[14] Shakespeare referred to the disease as "measles, which we disdain." Measles was usually seen as less troublesome than other diseases such as smallpox and leprosy. This can be seen in the use of the word "measly" to mean "small," "petty," or "trivial."[15]

Over the next few centuries, Europe continued to experience epidemics of measles every few years. Some were worse than others. The pattern of epidemics and the problems they caused seemed to change as the disease established itself over time. In the beginning of the eighteenth century, epidemics became more common, occurring every three years, often with deadly results. But during the middle of the century, very few people died from the disease. By the end of the century, measles epidemics were breaking out every other year, and measles became one of the most common causes of death among children.[16] In the twentieth century, measles had less of a devastating effect in Europe because there was a better standard of living and people were healthier.[17]

Measles in the New World

Whenever a group of people encounters a new disease that has never affected that group before, the disease can cause serious problems. This was certainly the case when Europeans brought measles to the New World.

When the Spanish conquistador Hernando Cortés arrived in Mexico, there were nearly 30 million people living there. By 1568, less than 50 years after Cortés's arrival, the population of central Mexico had shrunk to 3 million. By 1620, the population was reduced to 1.6 million. Similar drastic reductions occurred among native populations in many parts of the Americas. Smallpox and measles brought by the invaders played a major role in wiping out the native inhabitants.[18]

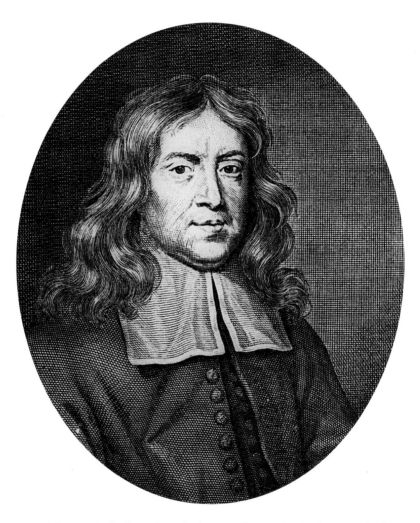

Dr. Thomas Sydenham described a measles epidemic that struck the people of London around 1670.

In the Americas, the early colonists believed that the diseases that often ravaged the native populations were just a sign that Divine Providence was on their side. It helped them to justify their conflicts with the Native Americans as they took over more and more of the land in the New World.[19] Of course, they—and earlier waves of colonists and explorers—were the ones who had brought the diseases in the first place. But they did not know that.

Measles in North America

Measles affected North America differently from Europe. The frontier was huge, and people were spread out. Immigrants came in waves from Europe, bringing with them diseases such as measles. So epidemics did not happen as often, but they were severe when they occurred, and affected people of all ages, not just young children.[20] Eventually, the distance between communities decreased, as the population increased and travel became easier and more common. The opportunity for disease to spread increased, too.

The first measles epidemic in the thirteen colonies occurred in Boston in 1657. The next one in Boston did not occur until thirty years later. But by the beginning of the nineteenth century, the pattern of measles epidemics in America was similar to that of Europe: Epidemics were breaking out every three years or so, and the disease was widespread, especially among children.[21]

More Knowledge, More Power

At the end of March in 1846, a workman from Copenhagen, Denmark, landed on the Faroe Islands in the North Atlantic. On April 1, he came down with measles. The islands had not had a measles case in sixty-five years, so anyone under sixty-five was not immune to the disease. By October, 6,100 of the 7,864 island inhabitants had developed measles, and 102 people died.

The Danish government sent a young doctor, P. L. Panum, to deal with the epidemic. Much of what we know about measles we have learned through Dr. Panum's careful observations. He confirmed earlier reports that measles was transmitted only by direct contact with someone who was actively ill. He determined that the best way to control an epidemic was to isolate the people who were ill. He also found that after exposure, there is a thirteen- to fourteen-day *incubation period* before symptoms develop. During this time, the person may feel well but can still transmit the disease to others. Dr. Panum noticed that no one over the age of sixty-five came down with measles and realized that the older islanders had become immune to the disease during the last epidemic. He concluded that people who recover from measles acquire a lifelong protection from the disease. This conclusion was confirmed thirty years later, when another measles epidemic swept the Faroe Islands. In that epidemic, no one over thirty came down with the disease.[22]

DEATH CAME
TO THE ISLANDS

Measles struck Hawaii for the first time in 1848, carried by settlers from California. In the epidemic that swept through the islands, one hundred fifty thousand natives became ill. More than a quarter of them died. In 1875 an epidemic in the Fiji islands was started when some British sailors with measles were allowed to land on one of the islands. Within three months, thirty thousand to forty thousand natives had died—close to a quarter of the entire population. From the Fiji islands the disease spread to other islands in the South Pacific, with equally devastating results. White men also brought tuberculosis and syphilis to the islands. Together these diseases reduced the native population in the South Pacific to only one tenth of the number who had lived there a century before. Greenland was more fortunate when a single case of measles in 1951 started an epidemic that swept through the forty-three hundred people who had never been exposed to the disease. Within six weeks, all but five of them had caught it. By that time, though, better medical care was available, and only 1.8 percent of the victims died.[23]

At the time when Dr. Panum made his observations, no one knew what caused measles—or any other infectious diseases. It was not until 1862 that Louis Pasteur proposed that diseases transmitted from one person to another were caused by microscopic germs. These germs invaded the body and attacked its tissues. Following up on this theory, Pasteur and other researchers soon discovered bacteria swarming in the body fluids and tissues of people and animals with various diseases. But the best microscopes of the time were not powerful enough to show viruses, so scientists were reluctant to believe that any microbes smaller than bacteria could exist.

In the late 1890s, it was established that some diseases were caused by viruses—germs so small that they passed through the finest filters used to trap bacteria. About that time, an American pediatrician named Henry Koplik was making careful observations of his young measles patients. He discovered that a day or two before the typical red rash appeared on the person's face and body, small red spots with blue-white centers appeared inside the mouth, in the linings of the cheeks. These spots are now called *Koplik spots*, although they had actually been noticed a century earlier by doctors in Jamaica and Maine.[24]

The first effort to protect people from measles dates back to 1758. An English physician, Francis Home, tried to immunize people against measles by injecting them with matter from patients' sores. But his crude attempts at immunization were not very successful.[25] In 1911, researchers produced typical measles symptoms in monkeys by injecting them with filtered material from human measles patients. In the late 1930s, researchers were finally able to grow measles viruses in tissue cultures outside the body, but standardized culture methods were not available until a decade later. In 1954, measles viruses were isolated by Nobel Prize–winning microbiologist John Franklin Enders and his coworkers. Over the next few years his research team developed methods for growing the virus in large quantities in chicken embryo tissues. By 1963, vaccines produced from killed or modified measles viruses had been tested and were available for general use.[26]

German Measles

Early Arabian physicians wrote about *al-hamikah*, a mild contagious disease with a red rash. They believed it was a form of measles, but today's medical historians think these were the first written descriptions of rubella. It was not recognized as a separate disease until the mid-1750s, when its symptoms were described by two German physicians, De Bergen and Orlow. For the next century there was so much interest in the disease among the German medical community that the rest of the world began to refer to it as "German measles." (The Germans called it *Rötheln*.) A Scottish physician, H. Veale, suggested the name *rubella* in 1866, in a paper describing thirty cases of the disease. In 1881 the International Congress of medicine in London decided that rubella was definitely a separate disease, although it was rather similar to measles. It was not realized

25

until the early 1940s that this mild disease could cause serious birth defects if it was caught by a pregnant woman.

Meanwhile, Japanese researchers V. Y. Hiro and S. Tasaka demonstrated in 1938 that rubella could be transmitted by injections of filtered nasal washings and therefore must be caused by a virus. The virus was isolated in 1962, which made it possible to develop a vaccine to prevent rubella.[27]

3

What Is Measles?

Ken's mother was getting worried. Her twelve-year-old son had been sick before, but this time was the worst she had ever seen. At first it had seemed like an ordinary sore throat. A throat culture, taken at the doctor's office, was positive for strep throat, so the doctor had prescribed penicillin. But after two days the antibiotic did not seem to be working. Ken was still coughing and running a fever of 102 degrees Fahrenheit. During the next few days the fever rose even higher, and then Ken developed a red rash on his face and body. The doctor thought Ken might have scarlet fever, or was perhaps experiencing a reaction to the penicillin, and prescribed a different antibiotic. But neither the rash nor the fever went away, and Ken complained that the light hurt his eyes. He was so groggy that he even walked into a mirror. "If he hadn't been immunized, I would think he had measles,"

Ken's mother remarked, thinking back to her own case of measles back in the 1950s. It turned out that she was right. The fever finally went down a few days later, but by that time some of Ken's classmates were developing the same kinds of symptoms. The 1989 measles epidemic had begun.[1]

Ken was miserable for a week or two, but then he recovered fully. Some of the victims of that epidemic were not so fortunate. Ten-year-old Hector, for example, seemed to have just a cold at first. But when he began to have difficulty breathing, he was rushed to the hospital—and died two days later. He had been immunized against measles before starting school, but apparently one shot was not enough. One-year-old Carrane was not due for a measles shot yet when the epidemic struck. Apparently the immunity she had received from her mother before birth had worn off, and she came down with measles. Then she developed pneumonia, and after five weeks on a respirator she died. Twenty-nine-year-old Frank apparently caught measles in the hospital, when he went to the emergency room to have a broken bone set. He, too, developed pneumonia and died. His mother could not remember whether he had ever been immunized against measles.[2]

A Viral Disease

The medical name for measles is *rubeola*. This name sounds similar to *rubella*, the medical name for German measles, a different disease that produces similar but milder symptoms. Both terms come from *ruber*, the Latin word for "red." Measles is sometimes called hard measles, or red measles (for the red rash it produces). It is also called *morbilli,* and the virus that causes it belongs to the genus *morbillivirus.*

Like other viruses, the measles virus is just at the borderline between the living and nonliving worlds. From 100 to 250 nanometers (less than ten millionths of an inch) in diameter, it consists of a core of RNA (a form of nucleic acid that contains all the instructions for infecting hosts and making new viruses) surrounded by proteins and lipids. It "comes alive" and can reproduce only within a living cell. When the measles virus comes in contact with a suitable host (usually a human being, although measles can infect monkeys in the laboratory), it attaches itself to the outer membrane of a host cell and gets

CONFUSING NAMES

Morbilli, a common name for measles, comes from the Italian *morbillo,* meaning "little disease." (Bubonic plague was referred to as *il morbo.*) The great Middle English writer Geoffrey Chaucer wrote about "mesel," but he was talking about leprosy. In the sixteenth century, many writers mentioned "small poxe and mesels" as though it were a single disease. Even by the eighteenth century, a diagnosis of "measles" or "morbilli" often meant that the person had scarlet fever, while a diagnosis of "scarlet fever" referred to diphtheria.[3]

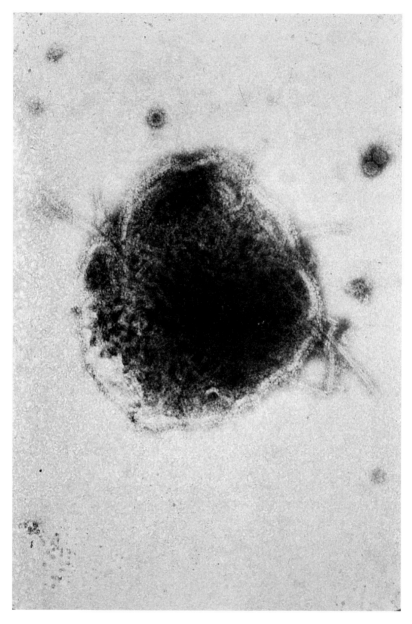

The measles virus.

inside it. There, like an uninvited guest, the virus takes over. It uses the host cell's raw materials for its own purposes and directs the mass production of new virus particles.

Usually measles viruses enter their human hosts when a person breathes in air containing droplets of moisture breathed out (or coughed out) by someone infected with measles. The moist membranes that cover the eyes and line the eyelids may also be an entry route. The delicate cells in the linings of the respiratory passages are the first to be attacked. Measles viruses settle in and multiply, and some of the lining cells become quite abnormal. Cells join together, forming many giant cells, sometimes with a hundred nuclei or more.[4] (Normal cells have only a single nucleus.) The infection quickly spreads to the tonsils and nearby lymph nodes.

The Body Defends Itself

The first cells that are attacked by a virus are unable to defend themselves. But several hours before an infected cell releases the new viruses it was ordered to create, a substance called *interferon* is released into the fluids surrounding the cell. This chemical tells neighboring cells to make an antiviral protein that will fight off viruses. When the virus attacks alerted neighboring cells, they are able to disobey the virus's orders. In many viral diseases, interferon helps delay the spread of infection, but it is not very effective in an early measles infection.

An hour or so after a virus invasion, cells in the nasal lining secrete extra mucus, a sticky fluid that helps to trap viruses. *Inflammation*—swelling, pain, heat, and redness—also

31

develops around the area of infection. These changes help to slow down virus reproduction, while making it easier for white blood cells, the body's disease fighters, to move around.

The chemicals released by virus-damaged cells act as distress signals, calling in several kinds of white blood cells. Some destroy invading germs before they can infect cells. Others are able to recognize foreign chemicals, such as the proteins on the outer coat of a virus. Some white blood cells produce *antibodies*, proteins that contain mirror images of the virus proteins. Antibodies attach to viruses, preventing them from attacking their target cells and making them easier for body defenders to destroy.

Once a person has antibodies that protect against a particular virus, his or her body will be able to prevent future infections by it—the person has become *immune* to that disease. Some of these antibodies continue to circulate in the blood for years, ready to defend against attacks by the same type of virus.

It generally takes about two weeks to make an adequate supply of antibodies to fight a virus the body has never met before; during that time the viruses multiply while the body's less specific defenses try to keep them in check.

Not a Fun Disease

Measles may have once been a very common childhood illness, but as experts like Dr. Lawrence D. Frenkel, director of the division of immunology, allergy, and infectious disease at the University of Medicine and Dentistry of New Jersey, point out, it is "one of the most severe" of all childhood diseases.[5] Children and young adults who get measles can become very ill.

Measles symptoms usually appear in two stages. About ten days after being exposed to someone with measles, signs of the first stage begin to develop. The patient feels tired and sick all over, with a slight fever and a runny nose and cough. The eyes are red, watery, and sensitive to light. The fever continues to rise each day. From three to seven days after the first symptoms develop, a blotchy red rash appears on the face and spreads over the rest of the body, while the fever soars to 103 to 105 degrees Fahrenheit.[6]

Stage 1: Respiratory Problems
Doctors talk about the "Three C's" of measles symptoms: cough, conjunctivitis, and coryza.

Cough: Measles can cause a severe, "brassy" cough, which usually begins early in the illness and lasts for up to ten days. This cough is caused by the virus attacking the lining of the trachea and bronchi, the breathing passages leading down into the lungs.

Conjunctivitis: Measles almost always causes conjunctivitis (pinkeye), an inflammation of the membrane covering the eyes. It does not affect vision, but it causes a redness and watering of the eyes. There may be pain in the eyes, and they also may be sensitive to light.

Coryza: Measles causes severe irritation in the nasal passages, which produces a runny nose (coryza). This lasts from the second to the fifth or sixth day.

Stage 2: Measles Rash

When you think of measles, the first symptom you think of is a rash. However, the telltale rash on the skin is not the first kind of rash that develops during measles. Shortly after the illness begins, small blue-white spots surrounded by red rings appear in the mouth, on the inside of the cheeks. These *Koplik spots* occur only in measles, and they occur in almost every case.

A few days after the Koplik spots appear, the skin begins to break out in the familiar measles rash. As this red rash appears, the Koplik spots fade.

The rash starts as slightly itchy, blotchy, pale red, flat sores. They first appear behind the ears and at the edges of the face. Soon the rash spreads to the forehead and face, and then down the body to the neck, trunk, arms, and legs. The spots become slightly bumpy. As the rash spreads down the body, the earliest spots join together, forming larger, deeper red areas. These large spots may bleed. While the rash is spreading, the fever rises to as high as 105°F (41°C).

The rash spreads all over the body within two or three days. By the time the rash reaches the feet, the patient's fever drops, and the runny nose and cough disappear. Soon the rash begins to fade, leaving a brownish stain that remains for a while. In areas where the rash was especially bad, the skin may begin to peel. In most cases the disease has run its course, and the patient is on the way to complete recovery.

Medical experts are not sure whether the measles rash is directly caused by the measles virus or not. There is evidence to suggest that it is the body's response to the virus—part of an

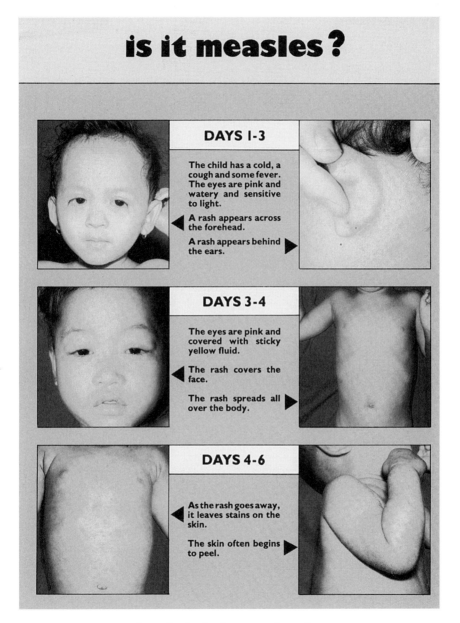

Stages in the development of measles.

immune response that clears away virus-infected cells. Children whose body defenses are not up to par, for example, do not develop the rash.[7]

Measles Complications

Measles can make a person feel very sick, but in most cases it clears up by itself after a week or ten days. However, more than one out of every twenty people infected with the measles virus develop complications.

Measles is most severe in infants and adults, as well as in people with an impaired immune system. In these populations, there is also a greater risk of dangerous complications such as ear infection, pneumonia, diarrhea, seizures (jerking or staring spells), brain damage, and even death.[8]

Measles by itself is not what causes most of the life-threatening complications. It can, however, lower a person's resistance, allowing bacterial infections, including ear, sinus, and lung infections (pneumonia), to occur.

In about one in a thousand cases of measles, the virus causes an inflammation of the brain called *encephalitis*.[9] This can be quite serious, causing hearing loss, convulsions, hyperactivity, learning disabilities, mental retardation, paralysis, coma, or even death.

In another rare but serious complication, the patient develops a dark purple skin rash. This is caused by bleeding due to a loss of platelets (disk-shaped structures in the blood that help it to clot). If a pregnant woman develops measles, there is a greater chance that she will die or have a miscarriage, premature labor, or an infant with a low birth weight.[10]

Typically, about one in one thousand patients with measles dies from complications. During epidemic outbreaks the number can be much higher. In the 1990 outbreaks, for example, the death rate was more than three times as high.[11]

Measles is not fatal to most American children who catch it, but each year it kills more than a million undernourished children in poor countries, especially in Africa.[12] Some experts think measles contributes to malnutrition, by causing a loss of protein from the intestines. Malnutrition makes people less able to fight off infections.

Atypical Measles

Some people who were immunized before 1968 received a vaccine that was made from an inactivated virus. When these people are exposed to the measles virus, some develop an unusual—"atypical"—form of measles. The rash in atypical measles is most often found on the arms and legs rather than the face and body. Complications may include lung inflammation and swelling of the hands and feet due to retention of fluids in the tissues.

Spreading Measles

Once you recover from measles, you usually do not have to worry about ever catching it again. (Proper vaccinations also protect you.) But measles has a way of finding those who are

MEASLES, WHEEZLES, AND SNEEZLES . . .

In A. A. Milne's tales about Winnie the Pooh, Christopher Robin comes down with the wheezles and sneezles and everyone wonders "If wheezles Could turn into measles, If sneezles Would turn Into mumps."[13] Some researchers think that measles may indeed turn into another illness. Studies have found a link between measles and Crohn's disease, a painful intestinal illness that affects two hundred fifty thousand young adults in the United States alone.

Swedish researchers found that people born during the peaks of five measles epidemics in central Sweden between 1945 and 1954 had a 46 percent greater chance of developing Crohn's disease than people in the area who were born at other times during that decade. In addition, other investigators found measles virus particles in the intestines of some Crohn's patients. Researchers believe that the measles virus may infect cells in a person's gut at an early age and remain there, but it does not cause problems until the person gets older and the immune system changes. Heredity may also play a role.[14]

not protected, because it is extremely contagious. How contagious? "[O]n a scale of one to 10 [measles is] pretty close to a 10," says Dr. Brad Hersh of the Centers for Disease Control and Prevention (CDC) in Atlanta, Georgia.[15] Even the slightest contact with an infected person can be enough to infect someone who is susceptible.

The measles virus can survive for only a few hours outside of a human body, but this is more than enough time for it to spread. A person may become infected in a room three hours after the carrier has left![16]

Measles is usually spread when someone comes into contact with nasal or throat secretions of infected people. Little children with runny noses often wipe their noses with their

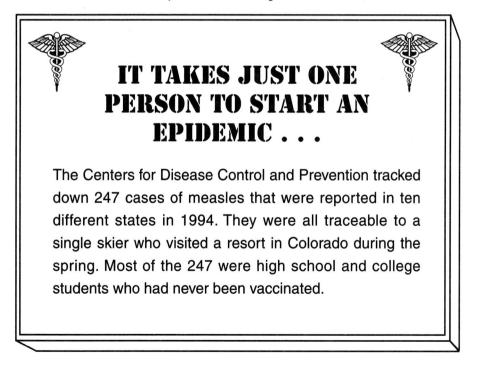

IT TAKES JUST ONE PERSON TO START AN EPIDEMIC . . .

The Centers for Disease Control and Prevention tracked down 247 cases of measles that were reported in ten different states in 1994. They were all traceable to a single skier who visited a resort in Colorado during the spring. Most of the 247 were high school and college students who had never been vaccinated.

hands and then touch toys or other children. The measles virus may also be spread when someone inhales airborne droplets that were coughed or sneezed out by an infected person.

Measles outbreaks usually occur in the winter and early spring. Those are the times of year when people tend to spend a lot of time indoors with the windows closed. Under such conditions, people literally breathe each other's air, which may be filled with germs. Since the winter and spring are part of the regular school year, children spend many hours a day together in classrooms, creating the perfect conditions for spreading measles and other respiratory diseases.

A parent whose child has measles usually knows to keep that child out of school or day care, but a child can be contagious during the incubation period, before any symptoms appear. A person with measles can spread the disease from five days before to five days after a rash appears.[17] By the time the skin starts to peel, there is no longer any danger of transmitting the virus.

Who Gets Measles?

In November 1985, a single preschooler came down with measles in a Jersey City, New Jersey, day-care facility. By June, more than nine hundred cases of measles had been reported in Jersey City, and thirty cases of pneumonia and one case of encephalitis had developed.[18] Before measles immunizations were available, epidemics often occurred every two to three years in any particular urban community.[19] In smaller communities outbreaks occurred less often, but they were more severe. Across the continent, there would typically be an epidemic, somewhere,

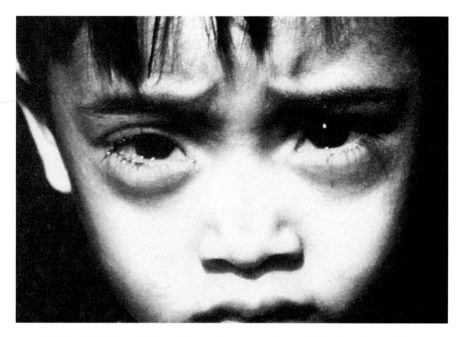

This child is suffering from the type of eye infection that often accompanies measles.

every year. Before the mid-1960s, 90 percent of Americans developed measles before they reached the age of twenty.

Children have always been most affected by measles. Now that most school-age children are vaccinated against the disease, it most commonly strikes preschoolers. Usually, if a mother has had measles or is immune through vaccination, a newborn baby will receive antibodies from the mother while in the womb. These antibodies protect the baby for the first four or five months or more. Most schools require that a child be vaccinated against measles before he or she enters school, at age five or six. Because of financial concerns, misinformation about vaccines, and lack of convenient access to immunization, many parents, particularly in inner-city neighborhoods, do not have their children vaccinated until it is time for them to enter school. But that leaves a big gap of time when the children are vulnerable—especially the children in preschool and day-care programs.

In recent years, measles outbreaks have also occurred in another population: among teens and college students who have previously been vaccinated but whose immune protection has weakened over time.

Measles Goes to College

Amy Lindemann, a Rutgers University junior, felt awful just before spring break in 1994. "I was sicker than a dog," she said. "I had a 104 degree fever. I was wearing about three sweaters and I was freezing cold." She did not realize at the time that she had measles. When she went home, she carried the germs with her. Soon her two sisters also came down with measles, even though they had both received measles shots as babies. What a way to spend a vacation! "It was a nightmare," the New Jersey college junior declared.[20]

Amy was not the only college student to develop measles that year. In 1994, 14 percent of all measles cases were due to outbreaks on college campuses, according to the CDC.[21] The college population was vulnerable because many of the students had received one dose of vaccine, before it was learned that a single shot may not protect everyone reliably. (At least thirty-nine states now require children to receive a second measles shot before age twelve.)

In a college setting, diseases can spread like wildfire. The students "eat together, they socialize together. They do everything together," Dr. Robert Bierman, Rutgers's director of student health services, points out.[22] When measles goes to college, there is even more cause for concern than when outbreaks occur in day-care centers or grade schools. Measles is more dangerous for college-age students than it is for young children, and it is more likely to bring on complications.

4

Diagnosing and Treating Measles

In an article in *Discover* magazine, Dr. Elisabeth Rosenthal describes how baffled she and other doctors and nurses were in 1989 when a very sick twenty-five-year-old was brought into their hospital's emergency room. The patient had spent three days in bed with a runny nose, sore throat, headache, and cough. He got a high fever; his pulse was racing; his watery eyes ached; his lymph nodes were enlarged; and he had a rash all over his body.

The senior resident doctor, Alex Martin, examined him first. "This guy looks terrible, but I have no idea what he has," he remarked. He asked Dr. Rosenthal to take a look. Both doctors were puzzled. They called a dermatologist (a skin doctor) and an infectious-disease specialist to help them diagnose the illness. Meanwhile, they checked their medical books and realized it might be measles. Like most United States doctors

44

in the late 1980s, they had never seen a patient with this once common childhood illness. The patient became the center of attention as doctors from all around the hospital came to see what a case of measles looked like, and brought in medical students to observe the rash firsthand.[1]

Confirming a Measles Diagnosis

Measles is very hard to diagnose during the first stage because the symptoms it produces are the same as those of a common cold. When the skin rash appears, diagnosis is much easier. The typical pattern of spots, combined with the other symptoms, usually helps a doctor to rule out other rash-producing diseases such as roseola infantum, German measles (rubella), or scarlet fever. Special tests are not usually needed, but there are a number of laboratory tests that can be used to verify the presence of the virus.

In the lab, a mucus sample from the throat or nose, or a blood or urine sample, might be tested for the presence of measles antigen (the characteristic protein found on the outside of the virus). Blood tests for measles-specific antibodies can help to confirm the diagnosis. Such antibody tests are also useful for screening large groups of people during a measles outbreak, when it is necessary to determine who needs to be immunized.

No "Cure" for Measles

There are no medicines available to cure measles once it develops. In spite of rapid advances in the development of antiviral drugs during the past thirty years, this is true of many viral diseases. In most cases the disease will run its course, and a person will have immunity against any further attacks.

Therefore, the main emphasis in treating measles patients is on keeping them as comfortable as possible while the body's defenses battle the invading germs. Keeping patients' strength up is also important for preventing dangerous complications. For this reason, doctors recommend that patients get plenty of bed rest and drink lots of fluids.

Treating the Symptoms

Many of the early symptoms of measles are very similar to those of a very bad cold or flu. Unfortunately, cold medicines, cough syrups, and nose sprays do not help much with measles symptoms. The patients should be encouraged to drink plenty of fluids to prevent dehydration. Inhaling steam or humidified air may help reduce irritation in the respiratory tract. Dim lights or sunglasses will help make light-sensitive eyes more comfortable.

For the headaches and high fever, doctors may recommend taking acetaminophen or other fever-reducing medicines that do not contain aspirin. Fever is actually one of the body's defenses against germs, but when fever goes too high it can become harmful. Generating all that heat burns up a lot of calories—just when the patient is too listless to feel like eating. Very high fevers may also lead to convulsions (painful, involuntary contractions of the muscles). Aspirin is not recommended for children or young adults with viral illnesses,

46

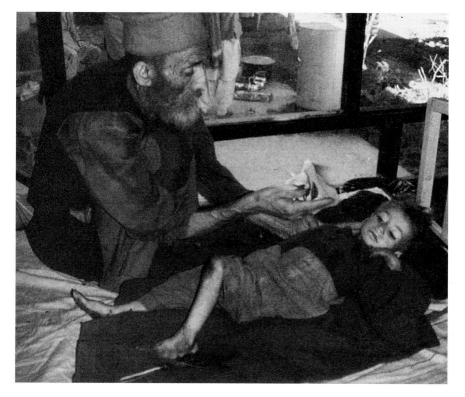

Bed rest is an important part of the treatment for measles.

because of Reye's syndrome. This is a rare but very serious illness, which has been linked with taking aspirin during viral illnesses.

What About Antibiotics?

Antibiotics are drugs that help the body to fight invading bacteria, but they are not effective against viral diseases like measles. However, antibiotics may be needed to treat secondary ear or lung infections that sometimes occur when measles weakens a person's immune system. (Because of the possibility of complications arising, a doctor should always be consulted whenever a child or adult comes down with measles.)

Antibiotics have actually been an important factor in the dramatic decrease in measles mortality that has occurred in the twentieth century, because most measles-related deaths are due to secondary infections. Penicillin and the other "wonder drugs" have not been the only factor in this drop, however. Children today are generally healthier and better nourished than in previous centuries, so their bodies are better able to fight off secondary infections. Sanitation and living conditions are also better, which reduces contact with germs that are potentially dangerous when the body is weakened.

Morale Problems

Measles makes patients feel so sick that all they want to do is stay in bed and not eat. However, they should be encouraged to drink liquids to prevent dehydration, and to eat to provide nourishment for fighting disease germs and repairing damage to the infected tissues. Soft foods may be easier for them to eat than a normal diet, since they require less effort and are less painful to swallow. Even though the eyes of measles patients may be very sensitive to light, it is important not to keep the room completely dark—this can become quite depressing. It is also not necessary to keep a child with measles isolated, away from contact with his or her brothers or sisters. Since measles is contagious well before any symptoms are visible, it is very likely that they will already have been exposed to the virus.[2]

As the measles patients' strength returns, they can gradually go back to normal activities. It is best to keep a child recovering from measles indoors, where play tends to be less physically exerting and there are fewer opportunities for contact with other people while the disease is still contagious.

The Vitamin A Link

According to a 1990 report in the *New England Journal of Medicine*, children with severe measles complications were not getting enough vitamin A in their diets. (Carrots, eggs, sweet potatoes, milk, and cantaloupes are rich sources of vitamin A.) The study was conducted in a large South African children's center. When the children were treated with vitamin A supplements, the measles-related death rate was cut in half, and children improved much more quickly than those who did not receive the vitamin.[3]

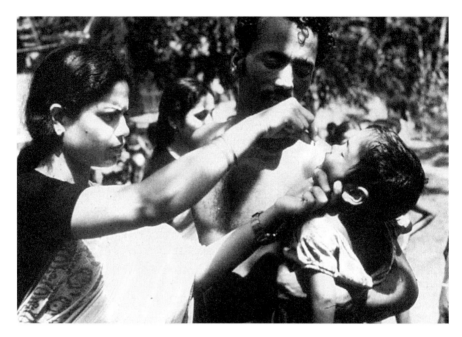

Studies have shown that children with severe complications from measles did not have enough vitamin A in their diets. Here, a health worker is giving a capsule of vitamin A to a child in a refugee camp.

For this reason, doctors may now prescribe megadoses of vitamin A for some children when they develop measles. In fact, according to the authors of the South African study, Dr. Gregory D. Hussey and Dr. Max Klein of the University of Cape Town, "all children with severe measles should be given vitamin A supplements, whether or not they are thought to have a nutritional deficiency."[4] However, large amounts of vitamin A should be taken only when prescribed by a doctor, because high doses of this vitamin can be toxic.

5

Preventing Measles

When New York State students came home from a statewide Key Club meeting in the Catskill Mountains in early spring 1992, some of them brought home more than they bargained for. A few weeks later, nine of these students, from all around the state, came down with measles.

One of these students was Peter, an honor student at a high school in Long Island. When he went to the doctor, health department officials notified his high school. The principal announced the news over the loudspeaker and cancelled the upcoming varsity baseball game and the Friday night dance. Meanwhile, Nassau County health workers contacted all of the people on Peter's paper route. Susan, a neighbor who had invited him into her house the previous Sunday while she wrote out a check, quickly scheduled an

51

appointment for her fifteen-month-old daughter to be vaccinated.

At Peter's high school, the county set up a free immunization program to inoculate any students who had not received two measles vaccinations. To ensure their participation in the inoculation program, the students would not be allowed to come back to school after spring break until they were vaccinated.

Meanwhile, state health officials sent warnings to each of the 123 schools that had had students attending the Key Club meeting, so that they could take extra precautions, too.[1]

Preventing Epidemics

There is no cure for measles, so the best approach is to prevent people from getting infected, by vaccinating them before they are exposed to the virus.

Vaccines are made from the kind of germ they are designed to protect against. Some vaccines are made from inactivated or killed viruses or bacteria. Others are made from certain products or parts of the invader, but not the whole disease germ. Many effective vaccines are made with live viruses or bacteria that are specially weakened so that they cannot cause disease in the body. Scientists have found, for example, that when measles viruses are grown for a long time in animal cells in a test tube, they gradually change and eventually become less able to spread in people and cause illness. Such weakened strains of germs are referred to as *attenuated.*

HOW VACCINES WORK

Vaccines trick the body into building up defenses against a particular disease-causing virus or other body invader without actually exposing it to the danger of disease. The vaccine contains look-alike chemicals that are similar to parts or products of disease germs. The immune system recognizes these chemicals as "foreign" (things that do not normally belong in the body), and therefore produces antibodies against them. These antibodies can also match up with parts of the real disease germs. So if measles viruses, for example, enter the body of a person who has received injections of measles vaccine, cells coated with antibodies floating in the person's blood quickly recognize the invader and neutralize it. These cells remember the antigen from the vaccination and mass-produce measles antibodies, which continue to attack the invading viruses and kill them before they can multiply to dangerous levels.

Problems with the Early Vaccines

Harvard researcher John Enders, who shared a Nobel prize with two of his colleagues for developing the basic methods for growing viruses in laboratory cultures, developed one of the first measles vaccines. It was a killed-measles virus vaccine, which was approved for general use in 1963, after five years of testing. This measles vaccine was used for only a few years, however, because it did not produce very high levels of protection, and the immunity was only temporary. Even worse, when people who had received the killed vaccine were exposed to measles virus years later, they were more likely to develop atypical measles. This was accompanied by serious complications such as pneumonia, fluid in the lungs, and swelling of the arms and legs.

There were different problems with the first live-measles vaccine, which was also approved for use in 1963. It had been attenuated by growing in animal tissues, but it often produced side effects of high fever and rash—almost as severe as the measles disease itself.[2]

In 1968 a more effective live-virus vaccine was introduced. This is the vaccine that is used today, but there were problems with it at first. If the vaccine is not properly stored in refrigerated containers, it loses its effectiveness. Studies by the CDC found that some high school students who were vaccinated with improperly stored vaccine later became infected with measles. In 1980 a stabilizing agent was added to the vaccine to help reduce the effects of temperature and exposure to light.

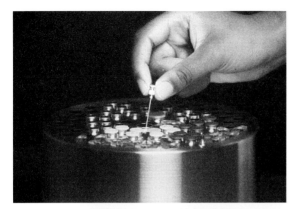

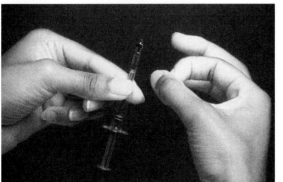

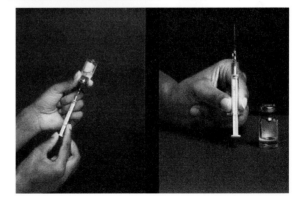

Vaccines for immunization must be carefully prepared and handled. Steps in the process include: putting a needle into the rack of a sterilizer (top); forcing air bubbles out of the syringe (middle); drawing vaccine from a bottle into the syringe (bottom).

Measles Vaccination Today

The measles vaccine is given by injection. It may be given by itself or combined with other vaccines, for example: measles-rubella (MR) vaccine or measles-mumps-rubella (MMR) vaccine. Usually the MMR form is used, except in young children from six to eleven months old.

In the United States most children receive the MMR vaccine at twelve to fifteen months of age. When there is an outbreak among children under one year of age, babies as young as six months may be vaccinated. Children who receive

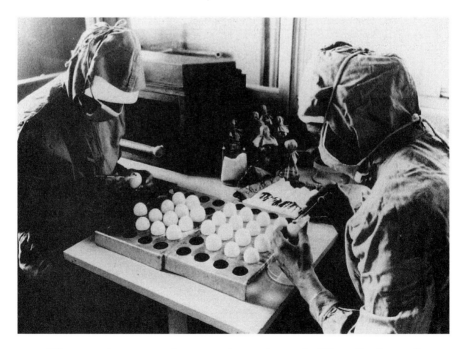

These people are preparing a measles vaccine at the Tirana Institute of Hygiene and Epidemiology in Albania.

a measles shot (MR) before one year of age should be revaccinated at fifteen months with MMR.

In developing countries in Africa and Latin America, where measles is still a major health problem, the World Health Organization recommends giving the vaccine at nine months of age. It may not be quite as effective when given that early, because some children still have protective antibodies from their mothers and therefore do not produce measles antibodies of their own. But health officials have found that if they wait much longer, many children have already been infected by the measles virus and developed the disease.[3]

Until 1989, the national health guidelines in the United States called for only a single dose of measles vaccine. But after the dramatic increase in the number of measles cases, the Immunization Practices Advisory Committee of the CDC changed its recommendations for measles vaccination. The committee suggested that children should receive a second measles shot before entering elementary school. (The American Academy of Pediatrics, however, recommends that children should not receive the second dose until eleven to twelve years of age, before entering junior high school.) The second dose is recommended as a safety net to immunize the 5 to 10 percent of children in whom the first vaccine was not effective.

Guidelines for Adults, Too

A second vaccination is also advisable for some adults, too. These include people who received only one measles shot, at

SMALLPOX SURVIVOR HELPS PREVENT MEASLES

"Why do children die of measles when a vaccine exists and the disease is preventable?" asked Ali Maow Maalin, a Somali hospital cook who had the world's last case of smallpox. In 1988 Maalin's little sister died from complications of measles. Her grieving family learned that they could have protected her against measles—and other killer diseases, too—by having her immunized. Maalin is determined to do his part to help others avoid the kind of tragedy that hit his family. The day after his sister was buried, Maalin went to the District Medical Office and volunteered to be trained to give immunizations. He speaks eloquently to the people of the district about the need for immunization. Maalin tells people how he survived smallpox, one of the world's oldest and deadliest plagues, which was finally wiped out completely through the dedicated efforts of health workers from all around the world. Sometimes people ask him why he is now putting so much effort into fighting "only measles." He answers,

> Because it killed my sister! Because it occurs so frequently! Because it spreads in the same way as smallpox and has a rash! And finally, if I succeed in convincing parents to protect their children against measles, then I can explain and also give the other immunizations that are available. First . . . I need the people's trust. I don't want them to lose a sister or a daughter before they discover too late that the child need not have died![4]

age twelve months. The CDC also recommends that anyone whose first dose of measles vaccine was given with immune globulin (an antibody-containing blood fraction given in the mid-1960s to lessen the side effects of the early live-virus vaccine) should receive two new doses of vaccine, at least a month apart.

When there is a measles outbreak in day-care centers, elementary schools, high schools, or colleges, the guidelines recommend that all school personnel born after 1956, as well as students and their brothers and sisters who are not immune, should be vaccinated. Usually students are required to show proof of having received two measles vaccinations (or other proof of immunity such as a measles blood test showing the presence of measles antibodies, or a doctor's diagnosis) before entering college.

Health-care professionals, especially those who work in hospital emergency rooms, are considered to be at high risk for coming in contact with diseases like measles. So all new health-care employees are required to show proof of immunity.[5] The Public Health Service recommends that all medical personnel born after 1956 should be revaccinated if there is a chance of their being exposed to the measles virus— medical workers born before 1957 have probably acquired the disease while working in medical facilities. Why 1957? That was the last big measles epidemic in the United States. Measles was so common before the vaccine that a person born before 1957 would have had the disease, or would have developed immunity to it.

Even when measles vaccine is given properly, about 4 to 5 percent of people remain unprotected or gradually lose their immunity. So, revaccination is also a good idea for anyone planning a trip to a developing country where the infectious disease rates are high.[6]

Refugee populations are susceptible to many dangerous diseases, and measles epidemics can be devastating, with high fatality rates. Mass immunization is important to prevent the spread of diseases like measles when tragedies cause refugees to flock together.

Side Effects

In some cases, side effects may occur from five to fourteen days after an injection of the current live-virus MMR vaccine. Serious or long-lasting problems are very rare, and the National Vaccine Injury Compensation Program provides compensation for people who are seriously injured by vaccines. There are risks involved in taking any medication. However, the possible risks from the measles vaccine are much smaller than the obvious problems that would occur if people stopped using it.

Who Should Not Receive the Vaccine?

There are a few groups of people who should not receive the MMR vaccine. Pregnant women should wait until after the baby is delivered. Those who are severely allergic to eggs or the antibiotic neomycin may have a reaction because the vaccine is

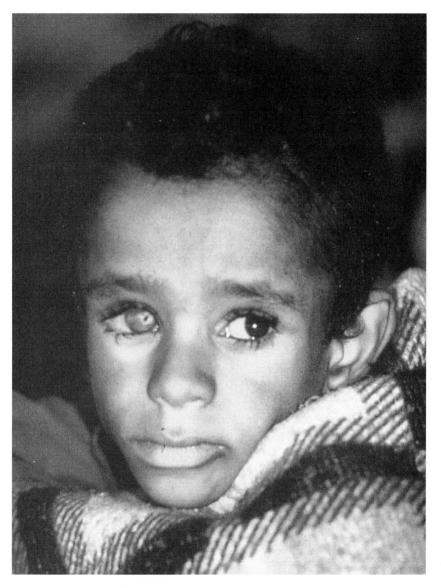

People living in refugee camps are especially susceptible to infections like measles. This child caught measles in a refugee camp in Sudan. Because no vitamin A was available at the time, his eyes were scarred by the infection.

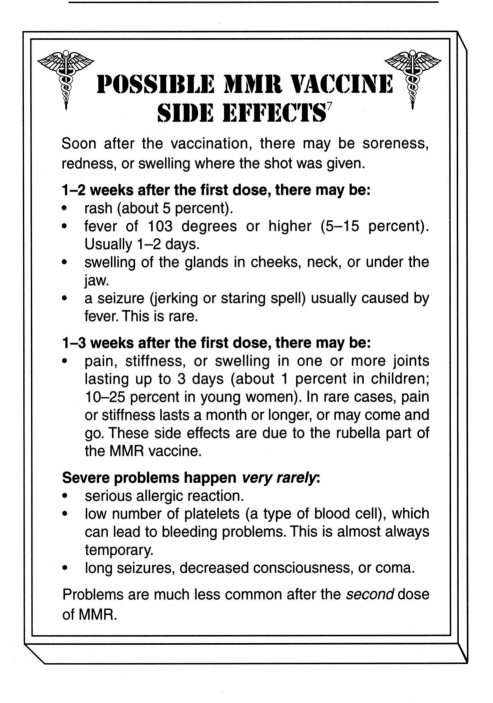

POSSIBLE MMR VACCINE SIDE EFFECTS[7]

Soon after the vaccination, there may be soreness, redness, or swelling where the shot was given.

1–2 weeks after the first dose, there may be:
- rash (about 5 percent).
- fever of 103 degrees or higher (5–15 percent). Usually 1–2 days.
- swelling of the glands in cheeks, neck, or under the jaw.
- a seizure (jerking or staring spell) usually caused by fever. This is rare.

1–3 weeks after the first dose, there may be:
- pain, stiffness, or swelling in one or more joints lasting up to 3 days (about 1 percent in children; 10–25 percent in young women). In rare cases, pain or stiffness lasts a month or longer, or may come and go. These side effects are due to the rubella part of the MMR vaccine.

Severe problems happen *very rarely*:
- serious allergic reaction.
- low number of platelets (a type of blood cell), which can lead to bleeding problems. This is almost always temporary.
- long seizures, decreased consciousness, or coma.

Problems are much less common after the *second* dose of MMR.

prepared using neomycin in a culture containing chicken embryo cells. Those with weakened immune systems due to illness or to drug or radiation therapy are also advised not to receive the vaccine.[8] (The CDC advises, and extensive experience confirms, however, that people infected with HIV generally *should* be vaccinated against measles; getting the disease would be much more dangerous for them than any side effects of the vaccine. They should be vaccinated early in the course of their illness, while they can still make protective antibodies.[9]) The tuberculin skin test for TB should be delayed until eight to twelve weeks after immunization with MMR or other live vaccines.

A 1991 report in the *Journal of the American Medical Association* noted that children who have bad colds when they get measles vaccinations may not be properly immunized against measles. (Their immune system is too busy fighting the cold germs to form good measles protection.)[10] Those who have received immune globulin or blood transfusions within the past few months should also postpone measles vaccination because the antibodies they received could block their own immune reaction.[11]

If You Are Exposed to Measles

A child or a young adult who is exposed to measles and is not certain about his or her vaccination status should be vaccinated within seventy-two hours of being exposed. The vaccine is less likely to be effective when given more than three days after exposure.[12] It is literally a race between the measles

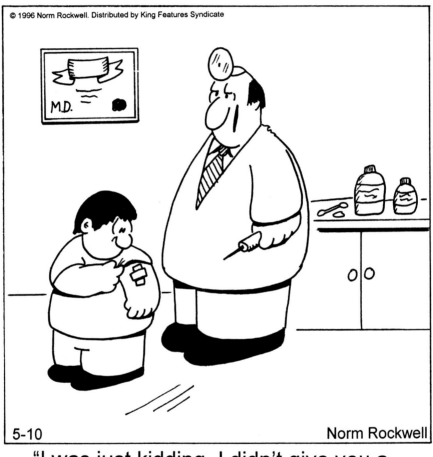

"I was just kidding. I didn't give you a tattoo. I gave you a measles shot."

virus's ability to multiply and the body's production of antibodies that could keep it in check. If the virus gets too much of a head start, the body cannot make enough antibodies to prevent illness.

But not everybody exposed to the measles virus realizes it in time to get vaccinated. The infected person may not have had any symptoms yet, or not everyone who was exposed may be notified promptly. Or there may not be enough time to get to a doctor within that narrow three-day window. Can anything be done in such cases to avoid developing measles after an exposure?

Before a measles vaccine was available, doctors sometimes gave people who had been exposed to someone with measles an injection of *gamma globulin* (a fraction made from human blood that contains many specific antibodies against disease germs) to help prevent the disease from developing. Gamma globulin provided temporary protection, helping the person to avoid developing the disease, or causing the disease to be less severe if it did develop. Today, gamma globulin may still be used in this way. It can help both those who did not find out that they were exposed to the disease in time to be vaccinated and those who should not be vaccinated for one reason or another.

Infants under one year of age who were exposed may be given a more specific antibody fraction, measles immunoglobulin (IG), because of the high risk of complications from measles in this age group. But there is a relatively narrow window for this form of prevention, too: measles IG is effective only when given up to six days after the exposure.

The immunization produced by injections of vaccine is called *active immunization*, because the person's immune system is actively involved, producing antibodies and other immune responses. Even after the threat of illness is over, some of the specific antibodies will be kept in reserve as "patterns" for mass-producing more antibodies if there is another attack by the same germ. But injections of immune globulin provide only temporary, *passive protection*. These antibodies were not produced by the person's own immune system (and in fact will prevent it from producing antibodies against the invading germ). They gradually disappear and are not replaced, because the immune system does not have a pattern on file to make more of them. So, health experts recommend that three months after receiving measles IG, a person should be vaccinated unless there is some strong reason not to. Otherwise, he or she could catch measles all over again.[13]

6

Measles and Society

The scene on a Chicago street was a familiar one in the summer of 1989. Salsa music blasting from the loudspeakers on the roof of a slowly moving car gave way to a voice that announced, "The Chicago Department of Health is offering free shots against measles at Roberto Clemente High School. Many cases have been reported in this area. Parents, please be sure your child is immunized." About nine hundred cases had already been reported in Chicago that year, and the city health officials were trying to get as many children inoculated as possible before the school term began. Five "measles mobiles" were spreading the word through the streets, and in neighborhood supermarkets, clerks were placing flyers in each bag of groceries. One young mother, who found a flyer in the envelope with her weekly paycheck, quickly took her two-year-old daughter to a clinic for a measles shot. "I didn't think of it until they started all this publicity," she said.[1]

The 1989 measles outbreak was a wake-up call for a nation that had grown a little careless in the effort against infectious diseases. "The potential is there in our inner-city populations for outbreaks of other diseases, including polio. Measles should sound the alarm," remarked Dr. Walter Orenstein of the CDC.[2] Chicago was only one of the cities that responded to the alarm. Health officials worked closely with local businesses to spread the word. In Los Angeles, for example, many companies included public service messages on the importance of immunization in their ads. Others donated a percentage of their sales to help fund the city's immunization program.

A Crusade that Fizzled Out

In 1978, after a worldwide campaign had succeeded in eliminating the threat of smallpox, Joseph A. Califano, Jr., then Secretary of Health, Education, and Welfare, announced a new goal for public health efforts: the elimination of measles from the United States by October 1, 1982. At the time, the goal seemed realistic. As the CDC pointed out, an effective vaccine was available, there was no animal host for the virus, and there were no measles "carriers" (people who carried the virus and could spread it to others without showing any symptoms of the disease).[3] It was just a matter of getting enough children immunized so that local outbreaks could not spread. Soon the virus would die out and disappear . . . or so it seemed.

Measles control efforts had already won some major victories. From prevaccine highs close to a million cases per year in the United States, the annual measles total was down to about fifty-seven hundred cases in 1977. A national Childhood Immunization Initiative, launched in the spring of 1977, aimed to immunize at least 90 percent of American children under the age of fifteen against a number of diseases for which vaccines were available (including diphtheria, pertussis, and polio in addition to measles) and to develop a permanent system to maintain that level of protection.[4] Joint efforts by federal and state officials helped to identify the children who needed vaccinations and set up means of ensuring that they would get them. By mid-1979, all fifty states required proof that a child had received all the necessary vaccinations as a condition for entering school. Thirty states had the same requirement for all students from kindergarten to the twelfth grade.

By 1980, 91 percent of all United States schoolchildren had provided proof that they had either had natural measles or had been vaccinated against it.[5] In the years that followed, the numbers got even better. At the beginning of the 1981–82 school year, 96 percent of children entering school in the United States had been vaccinated against measles, and in 1981 the total number of measles cases in the nation was down to 3,124. In addition to the immunization campaign, health officials closely monitored measles cases and clinics were set up, where children could get emergency vaccinations or booster shots when local outbreaks occurred. The national campaign did not make its target date—in 1982 there were 1,714 reported measles cases—but it looked like victory was only a matter of time.[6] In fact, the July-August 1982 issue of *FDA Consumer* magazine featured an article titled "How the Measles Virus Was Done In."[7]

In 1983 the measles total fell further, to 1,497. Unfortunately, after 1983 the number of measles cases began to go up again—first a little, and then a huge jump to about eighteen thousand cases in 1989 and close to twenty-eight thousand in 1990.[8]

What Went Wrong?

The campaign to conquer measles was partly a victim of its own success. As the numbers of cases plunged, people forgot how common (and how dangerous) measles used to be. So, increasing numbers of people did not bother to get their children immunized.

The situation was especially bad in the cities, particularly in the poorer, inner-city areas. In the 1989 outbreak, cases among unvaccinated preschool children in just three cities—Chicago, Houston, and Los Angeles—accounted for nearly 25 percent of all the measles cases in the nation![9] In Chicago, 75 percent of the 2,232 cases that year were in preschool children. There, and in other cities, it was found that only half of the mainly African-American and Hispanic children in inner-city schools had been vaccinated on schedule, compared to close to

80 percent of students in schools attended mainly by white children.[10]

Health experts have found five main reasons for low vaccination rates:

- *Cost*—Vaccinations can be expensive and may not be covered by health plans.
- *Access barriers*—Many people do not have regular health care, and clinics may not be convenient.
- *Ignorance*—Parents may not be aware of all the vaccinations needed.
- *Dysfunctional caregivers*—Immaturity, mental illness, or other problems may cause parents to neglect their children's health needs.
- *Missed opportunities*—Health-care professionals may not check a child's immunization records at an office or clinic visit.

Schoolchildren and college students who *had* been vaccinated also accounted for some of the new measles outbreaks. Some had been vaccinated with older, less effective vaccines. Others had received only a single dose, at too young an age to form effective immunity. In some cases the vaccine just did not work. It has a reported failure rate of 2 to 5 percent, and some health officials believe the actual rate could be as high as 10 percent.[11] "Five percent may not seem like a lot, but over a period of years, this adds up to thousands of adults who are not protected," points out Dr. William L. Atkinson, a medical epidemiologist at the CDC.[12] Moreover, some people who did produce effective antibodies after vaccination lose their protection over time. Ironically, the small number of measles cases in the United States and other developed countries may contribute to this loss. When measles is common in a population, people's immune systems are continually stimulated by exposure to the virus. But as immunization rates rise, there is less "wild" measles virus circulating, and a person is less likely to be exposed to it. Without the new stimulation, the patterns for making specific antibodies may gradually be lost.

Winning Again . . . Maybe

After the alarming measles outbreaks in 1989 and 1990, state and local health departments began major efforts to increase the vaccination rates among children. These efforts soon paid off. In 1993 there was a record low of 312 cases of measles, and many health officials were claiming a major victory. "We have seen measles virtually disappear in the United States in 1993," said Dr. William L. Atkinson of the CDC in Atlanta. "This would be the lowest total of measles ever reported in the United States since reporting began."[13] Another hopeful trend was the fact that the pattern of measles cases had changed. Before 1993, measles cases in the United States typically occurred among preschool children in cities. Since then, however, Dr. Atkinson noted, "We are no longer seeing those giant outbreaks in large cities. The largest outbreaks have all been in school kids, and the biggest we've seen is about 40 cases."[14]

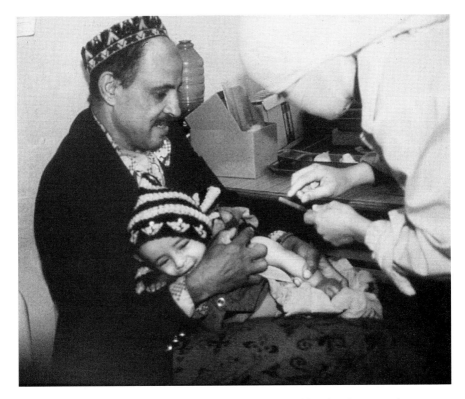

Both in the United States and all over the world, efforts are being made to prevent future measles epidemics. Here, a health worker is giving an MMR shot to a child in a clinic in a developing country.

A COLLEGE STATE
OF EMERGENCY

Early in 1994, a Rutgers University student brought back an unwelcome souvenir from a vacation in Spain: measles. By late March, twenty university students had developed the disease. The New Jersey Department of Health declared a measles emergency. This meant that state funds could be used to set up free immunization clinics at the health centers on three university campuses. Twenty-two thousand students, faculty, and staff were vaccinated over the next few weeks. But it was not easy to get people to go and get the free vaccinations. "Most students . . . just will procrastinate and not go exactly when you ask them to do it. If students know someone who has the measles then they consider it more of a real health threat," explained Marie Logue, a Rutgers college dean.[15] Thousands of letters were sent out. Volunteers and staff personally delivered messages to students who needed to be immunized. University health officials made it clear that those who needed vaccinations had better get them. Those who did not would not be allowed in class or in their dormitories. Grades, transcripts, and diplomas would also be withheld. "I just think it's an inconvenience," complained Adam Rypinski, a Rutgers college junior. "I have exams coming up." But he and his girlfriend went to get inoculated. "I think it's the right thing to do."[16] It was harder to get faculty and staff members to comply. Two days before the two-week vaccination program was to end, only 55 percent of the faculty had been vaccinated.[17]

At the same time the United States was experiencing an all-time low number of measles cases, however, Puerto Rico was suffering through a major measles epidemic. By 1994 the total for the small island territory had jumped to 958 measles cases.[18] By 1995, though, the number of cases of measles was again the lowest ever. In fact, late in 1995 the Pan American Health Organization reported that there had been only forty-five hundred measles cases that year in the whole Western Hemisphere—down from twenty-three thousand the year before. Of the forty-one countries of North, Central, and South America, twenty-one had no measles cases at all! These encouraging figures reflected a stepped-up effort to vaccinate children between nine months and fourteen years of age, whether they had been vaccinated before or not. As of the end of 1995, 93 percent of children in the Americas had been vaccinated against measles.[19]

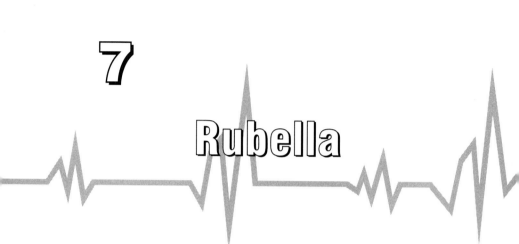

7

Rubella

I n the early 1940s, Dr. Norman McAllister Gregg, an ophthalmologist in Sydney, Australia, was confused by what seemed to be an epidemic of blindness among newborn babies. He was seeing an unusually high number of newborns with cataracts (a clouding of the eye lens that blocked their vision). Even more surprising, these babies seemed to be suffering from other birth defects as well, such as deafness, mental retardation, and heart defects.

Dr. Gregg interviewed the mothers of the babies and found that most had developed German measles during their pregnancy. Dr. Gregg published his findings. At first the medical community would not accept the idea that German measles could be linked with such serious birth defects. In 1944, for example, experts wrote blistering editorials attacking his theory in *The Lancet*, a prestigious British medical journal.

For centuries doctors had thought that rubella was a rather mild disease that quickly passed and rarely caused problems. But other researchers soon found supporting evidence for Dr. Gregg's hypothesis when they looked at previous studies on birth defects.

New studies were begun in which researchers looked for women who had had rubella during pregnancy. They compared the frequency of birth defects for the babies of these women with those of women who had not had German measles during pregnancy—and found that there was a definite link.[1]

What Is Rubella?

Rubella is called *German measles* because of research done by German scientists. It is also sometimes referred to as *three-day measles* because, unlike regular measles, it passes very quickly.

The symptoms of rubella are somewhat similar to those of measles, but the virus that causes it is not related to the measles virus. German measles is caused by a virus in the genus *rubivirus*, which scientists have classified in the family Togaviridae. The rubella virus particles are spherical in shape, and fifty to seventy-five nanometers wide (about two to three millionths of an inch).

How Rubella Is Spread

German measles is passed along when susceptible people come in contact with discharge from an infected person's nose or mouth. They may breathe in airborne droplets from a cough

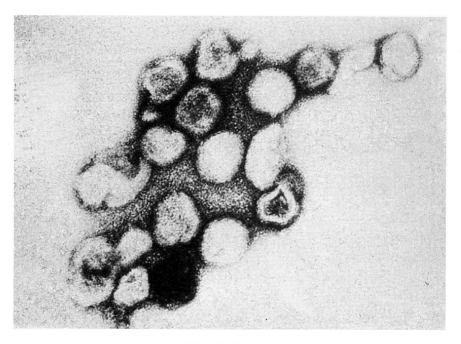

The rubella virus.

or sneeze, or touch surfaces contaminated with the virus. The virus then gets inside its victim when the person touches his or her nose, mouth, or eyes. Infection may also occur through contact with an infected person's blood, urine, or feces. Rubella is not as contagious as measles, and many people who are exposed to the virus do not become infected.

Once the rubella virus has entered the body, it begins to multiply in the upper respiratory tract. Then it is spread by local lymph nodes to the bloodstream. Two to three weeks after a person is infected with the rubella virus, the first symptoms develop. The incubation period can range from twelve to twenty-three days, but in most cases symptoms appear within

HE WAS REALLY MOTIVATED

Thomas Weller, a member of the Harvard University research team that won a Nobel prize for discovering how to grow polioviruses, went on to hunt down a number of viruses including the chicken pox virus, cytomegalovirus (a herpesvirus), and the rubella virus that causes German measles. He was highly motivated in his studies of the rubella virus—his own family was suffering from German measles at the time. In fact, the rubella virus that he grew in tissue culture came from his ten-year-old son! His discovery made it possible for a vaccine against German measles to be developed.[2]

sixteen to eighteen days. The disease is contagious for a week before symptoms appear, and for five to seven days after the characteristic rash develops.[3]

Who Gets Rubella?

German measles is an *endemic* disease (always present) everywhere in the world except in isolated communities, such as on remote islands. Until a vaccine was developed, large epidemics occurred regularly around the world. Before the vaccine was introduced in the United States, there were about sixty thousand recognized cases in the United States each year. Today there are only a few hundred cases per year.[4]

Like measles, rubella was once a widespread childhood illness, but the typical age for becoming infected was usually higher than for measles. Before vaccines were available, 20 percent of preschoolers had developed antibodies; 80 percent or more of seventeen- to twenty-year-olds had been exposed. Before 1969, major rubella outbreaks occurred in the winter and spring, every six to nine years, in the United States and other developed nations. In more remote communities, outbreaks occurred every ten to fifteen years.

Usually school-age children would get German measles and then it would spread readily within a family. Infants who are born to immune mothers are protected for six to nine months.

Rubella Symptoms

German measles usually causes mild symptoms, especially when it occurs in young children. Some people may not even realize they have it.

The first signs of illness are usually mild respiratory problems, such as a runny nose with reddened eyes, slight fever, and headache. Swollen glands behind the ears and in the neck may cause soreness and pain, and may persist for two to three weeks. The swollen "glands" are actually lymph nodes, which contain disease-fighting cells. The swelling is inflammation, one of the body's defensive reactions against invading viruses.

The day after the lymph nodes swell, a slightly itchy pink rash breaks out on the face. It quickly spreads down to the chest and stomach, and then down to the feet. The rubella rash is usually made up of small pink dots that remain separated, unlike the flat reddish-brown spots in measles that join together to form large blotches. It comes and goes rather quickly—usually in one to three days. By the time it breaks out on the trunk, the rash on the face may have already disappeared. At least half of those who develop German measles have such a mild case that they do not even develop a rash.[5]

Complications

Although rubella is usually a mild illness in children, complications can occur—especially in people who catch it as an adult. Nearly one third of adult women with rubella have joint problems (arthritis), which appear at the same time as the rash or shortly afterward. Painful swelling and redness may

81

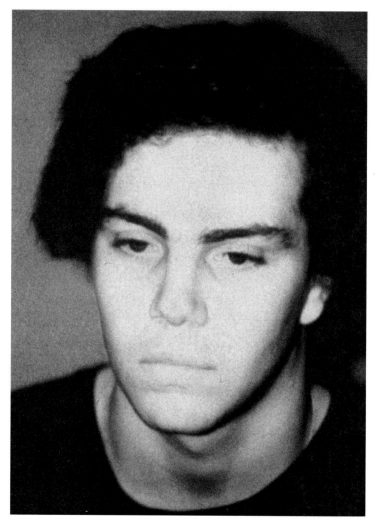

This young man's face shows the typical rubella rash.

develop in the finger joints, wrists, and knees. These problems may be mild, lasting for only a few days; or painful arthritis may last for months.

In rarer cases—about one in six thousand cases—German measles may affect the nervous system, producing high fever, convulsions, and other symptoms typical of encephalitis. Nearly 20 percent of children affected this way die, but the others usually recover completely.

Rubella can also lead to diseases that appear much later in life. One such disease is diabetes, in which the body is not able to use sugar properly.

Congenital Rubella Syndrome (CRS)

The most serious complications of German measles occur in unborn children. Before the MMR vaccine, pregnant mothers had serious reason to worry when their school-age children developed German measles. A woman who has never had rubella or a German measles vaccine and develops German measles during the first three months of pregnancy has a chance of developing serious problems. The mother may have a miscarriage, or the baby may be born prematurely, with congenital rubella syndrome (CRS). The many birth defects associated with this syndrome include: heart defects, liver infections, cataracts, deafness, bone damage, and mental retardation. More than half of the newborns whose mothers had rubella during the first three months of pregnancy are born with congenital rubella syndrome.[6] Severe symptoms may also be observed in about 5 percent of babies born to mothers who had rubella during the fourth month of pregnancy, but they rarely appear when the illness occurred later in the pregnancy.[7]

Infants born with congenital rubella syndrome can also infect other infants in the nursery as well as siblings at home, because they may continue to spread the rubella virus for months after birth. (Although antibodies against rubella are present in the bodies of both the mother and the baby, they apparently are not strong enough to clear the baby's body of the virus.)

Some medical experts believe that the rubella virus interferes with the normal growth of a fetus in the womb. Studies on fetal cells growing in laboratory culture dishes have found that infection with rubella virus slows down the rate of cell division. This effect could decrease the total number of cells, and thus explain the small size typical of rubella babies. The death of key cells or the slowing of their multiplication could also interfere with the formation of organs in the developing fetus, such as the heart, brain, eyes, and ears.

It has been estimated that the average cost of health care for just one person with CRS is more than $200,000. Before rubella vaccine became available, there were sixty to seventy cases of CRS in the United States each year. In 1989, twenty years after use of the vaccine was begun, only three cases of CRS were reported.[8]

Diagnosing Rubella

Diagnosing rubella on the basis of its rash may not be very reliable. Several other common childhood diseases have similar-looking rashes, and some people with rubella never

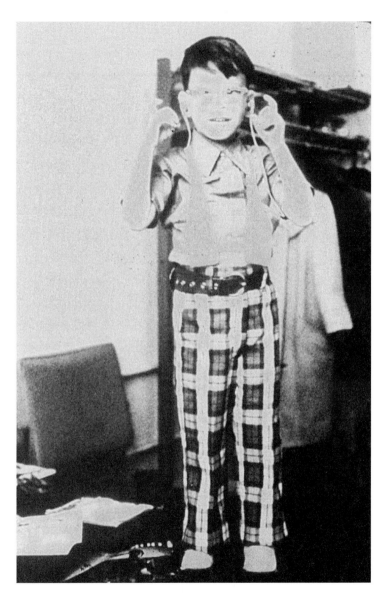

In this case, CRS resulted in deafness and mental retardation.

develop a rash at all. Yet there are some situations when it is important to know whether an illness is really rubella or some other viral disease. For example, a pregnant woman who is exposed to rubella or develops an illness with a rash may not remember whether she ever had the disease or the vaccine in childhood. Or doctors may need to know whether a child born with symptoms suggestive of CRS actually has the disease. (If so, the child could infect others with rubella.)

Blood tests can determine whether a person has ever had rubella, and whether an active infection is going on. More than twenty diagnostic kits have been developed to test for rubella antibodies. One type, rubella-specific IgG, indicates that the person has immunity to rubella. A sharp rise in the amount of rubella antibodies in two blood samples taken at least ten days apart indicates that the person has just had an active rubella infection. A different kind of rubella antibodies, belonging to a type called IgM, can also be a sign of an active infection, since these antibodies are produced in the first immune response to the invading virus. Unlike the IgG type, IgM antibodies are too big to pass from the mother's body into the bloodstream of a developing fetus. So the presence of rubella IgM in a newborn baby's umbilical cord blood is a sure sign of congenital rubella infection.[9]

Tests to confirm a rubella diagnosis may also be based on isolating the virus and growing it in culture. The virus can be found in blood serum and urine for a week before symptoms begin, but disappears soon after the rash appears. It continues to be shed from the nose and mouth for up to two weeks after

Reported Rubella—United States 1966–1993

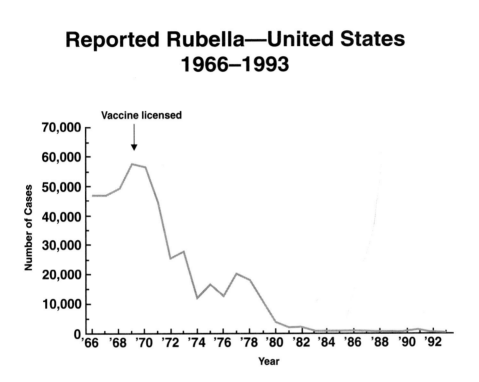

The development of a vaccine against rubella led to a sharp drop in the number of cases in the United States.

the rash begins.[10] Cell culture is not a routine method for diagnosing rubella, but it may be used to confirm cases of CRS.

Doctors are required to report all cases of rubella and congenital rubella syndrome, which helps to establish proper control measures. Any pregnant women who have come in contact with someone with rubella need to be identified and tested.

Treatment

A person with German measles is contagious and should avoid contact with others who have not been vaccinated or have not had the disease. Bed rest might be needed. Acetaminophen or other drugs to reduce fever or pain may also be prescribed.

Preventing Rubella

Like most viral diseases, the best treatment for German measles is to prevent it from occurring in the first place. Vaccines against rubella were developed in the 1960s and were approved for general use in 1969. Several strains of attenuated rubella virus have been developed, but only one (a stronger vaccine, licensed in 1979) is currently being used in the United States. Like the measles vaccine, it is made from a live, attenuated virus. It has been found to be 95 percent effective.

Today, a person usually receives a rubella vaccination in the same injection as measles and mumps vaccines. Side effects for the German measles vaccine are not common, but occasionally

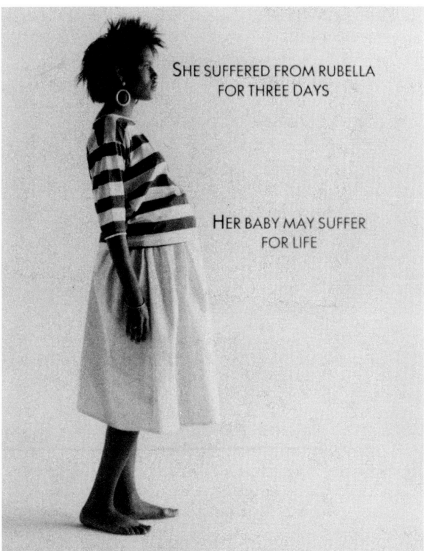

SHE SUFFERED FROM RUBELLA
FOR THREE DAYS

HER BABY MAY SUFFER
FOR LIFE

This woman didn't get vaccinated against Rubella. Now she's pregnant and she's caught the disease. Rubella won't have any lasting effect on her, but her baby may well be born deaf or blind or both. It may also suffer heart and brain damage. If only she'd been vaccinated before she became pregnant. It's so simple to avoid Rubella. So avoid it.

This is a poster warning women about the dangers of Rubella to their unborn babies.

it may cause fever, a slight rash, arthritis, or in extremely rare cases, shock.

Unlike the diseases for which most vaccines are developed, rubella is not a serious disease—except for babies in utero. Since the vaccine uses a live, attenuated virus, there is a small theoretical risk to the fetus; so, it is generally not given to pregnant women, and adult women who are given the vaccine are advised not to become pregnant for at least three months. However, studies of women who were inadvertantly vaccinated while pregnant have revealed that none have had any problems, and the majority of children born to these mothers are without rubella infection.

Vaccine Strategy

In the United States the strategy for rubella immunization has been to produce a *herd immunity.* If enough people are immune to a disease, then the virus will not be able to survive in the population because there are not enough susceptible people to keep the chain of infection going. So, in the United States, vaccination efforts have focused on immunizing young children.

Scientists have found, however, that even high levels of herd immunity are not always enough to prevent the spread of rubella in some communities.[11] So, there has also been an emphasis on vaccinating adolescent girls and adult women who have not previously developed immunity to rubella. The vaccine is recommended especially for female health-care workers and for teachers and young adults at colleges and

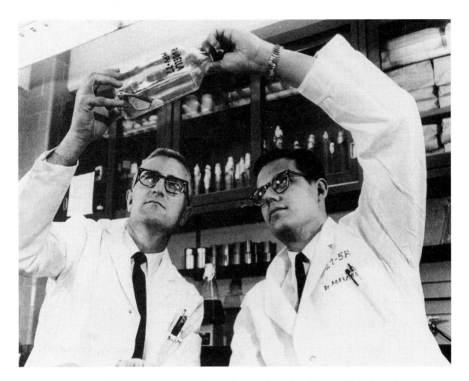

NIH researchers, Drs. Harry Meyer, Jr., and Paul Parkman, developed one of the first rubella vaccines. They are shown in 1967 holding up a culture of the HPV-77 rubella virus strain used in preparing the vaccine.

other types of institutions.[12] Mass immunizations are set up whenever there is an outbreak in a school.

Like other live-virus vaccines, rubella vaccine is not recommended for people with a weakened immune system or those taking immunosuppressive drugs. There is no harm in giving the vaccine to someone who is already immune, so doctors do not usually bother running laboratory tests before immunizing a young woman against rubella. In some countries, such as Australia, girls from eleven to thirteen years old are routinely given rubella shots without testing them for antibodies.[13]

In Australia and the United Kingdom, vaccination efforts have been targeted to teenage females, rather than to young children. The rationale behind this strategy is that natural infection may provide stronger and longer-lasting immunity than vaccines. So, they say, why interfere with the natural process by vaccinating young children? By doing so, we may be "protecting" them against a mild childhood illness while leaving them vulnerable to a more dangerous infection later. Immunizing young teenage girls ensures that their resistance will be high during the important childbearing years. In fact, their immunity will be strengthened by exposure to the wild virus that is still circulating in the community. In theory this strategy might seem more effective than herd immunity, but in practice it has not led to a decrease in either rubella or CRS, because the vaccination programs have missed many of the susceptible young women.[14]

8

Measles and the Future

In March 1993, the Children's Vaccine Initiative Committee met in a conference in Bellagio, Italy, to map out the best strategy for the continuing war against measles. At that time, the committee noted, measles vaccination programs were preventing more than 1.5 million deaths from measles in developing countries each year; yet about a million children were still dying each year from this preventable disease.

The committee discussed how further investments could best be used to strengthen the measles immunization programs and gain the knowledge needed to bring about more effective measles control. They recommended a three-part attack: 1) The use of the current live, attenuated vaccines should be improved and expanded. 2) Research and development efforts should be aimed at developing a better measles vaccine—one that is safe, is not neutralized by the mother's antibodies present in very young children, and does not need to be so carefully refrigerated. 3) A balanced investment program should include the development of the most effective vaccination strategies in each country and also more basic research to provide understanding of how the measles virus produces its effects and what caused the bad side effects of older measles vaccines.

Research efforts planned for the next decade should also include studies of the measles virus and differences between the wild and attenuated types and studies of factors that might protect against or promote severe measles (for example, nutrition and infections with other diseases, particularly AIDS). There is also an urgent need to develop a simple, rapid, and accurate diagnostic test that can be used in on-the-spot studies of measles outbreaks.[1]

Wiping out Measles: A Model Case

In November 1994, a Finnish team of scientists announced that the national immunization program had wiped out home-grown cases of measles, German measles, and mumps in Finland. "There are now fewer than thirty sporadic cases of each of the three diseases each year, and those are probably imported," the Finnish team reported in the *New England Journal of Medicine*.[2] Finland is the first country to wipe out these diseases through a massive immunization program. Since 1982, all children in Finland between the ages of sixteen months and six years have been vaccinated with MMR. Under the country's health-care system, the shots are given for free.

THE CASE OF THE MYSTERY DISEASE

In September 1994, real-life health scientists felt like they were starring in a science-fiction thriller. Fourteen racehorses died on a horse farm in Australia, and then their trainer died, too. The grisly symptoms included high fever, massive amounts of fluid in the lungs, and a bloody froth flowing from the nose. A medical team from Australia's top-security Animal Health Laboratory was called. A day later the medical team was testing samples taken from the dead and dying horses. They set up cultures to grow any viruses that might be present. Meanwhile, the team tested for various horse-disease viruses and bacteria and also for poisons such as insecticides. All the results were negative. By the fourth day after the outbreak, the tissue cultures began to show signs of a virus growing. An electron microscope revealed viruses with the herringbone shape typical of the morbilliform family, which includes the measles virus. But no known viruses in this family infected both horses and humans. The new virus was found in the lungs of several of the horses that died (and also in the kidneys of the dead trainer), but not in the lungs of healthy horses. When injected into healthy horses, the mystery virus made them sick. Next, the researchers mapped the virus's genetic "fingerprints." In just twelve days, the researchers had isolated and identified the first new member of the morbilliform family to attack humans since measles was first written about, in the ninth century.[3]

Dr. Michael Heisler of the Carter Center in Atlanta and Dr. Julius Richmond of Harvard Medical School wrote an accompanying editorial in the journal, declaring that the success in Finland could be a guideline to ridding the world of childhood diseases like measles. "With appropriate global leadership and political will, parents and children can be freed from fear of measles, mumps, rubella, and polio as well. Our colleagues in Finland have given us an example."[4]

Can We Still Wipe out Measles?

American health officials have seen their optimism about wiping out measles crushed several times. The United States is so much bigger than Finland. Do health officials still think measles can be eliminated here?

Most health officials believe that diseases like measles could be eliminated if the new CDC guidelines for childhood immunizations are strictly followed. If all children were to receive two injections of measles vaccine, for example, most of the cases of vaccine failure would be prevented.

However, there are major obstacles to overcome before the goal of immunizing everyone can be achieved. With the uncertain future of health care in our country, getting everyone vaccinated remains a problem. The budget passed by Congress in 1993 included a provision to provide free vaccines to all children whose vaccinations are not covered by health insurance. A 1995 report to Congress by the General Accounting Office (GAO) noted, however, that the cost of vaccines is not the main barrier to children's receiving all their needed immunizations on schedule. The GAO recommended that a better result could be achieved at a lower cost by specifically targeting the areas where immunization rates are still low, and by reducing missed opportunities for giving vaccinations through Medicaid programs, public health clinics, and other health-care providers who are already in contact with the underimmunized children.[5]

Looking for Better Vaccines

Health experts are also hopeful that better vaccines will be available in the future. In developing countries, measles in children less than a year old is a serious problem. These children are particularly vulnerable to deadly complications. The vaccine currently used is very reliable for adults and children fifteen months or older, but not very effective in younger infants.

In the early 1990s, health officials around the world were excited about a new experimental vaccine that seemed to be very effective in immunizing infants in the Third World. Worldwide, measles strikes about 44 million children a year and kills about 1.5 million children. Scientists thought the new vaccine could help reduce these horrifying statistics.[6]

The experimental vaccine was made with a special strain of measles virus that allowed it to be used in concentrations of ten to one hundred times the normal concentration. In preliminary trials in several countries, four- to six-month-old infants became immune to measles after vaccination. In 1990 the World Health Organization (WHO) recommended that this new vaccine (high-titer Edmonston-Zagreb vaccine) be used in other areas around the world where measles in younger infants is a major health problem.

The bubble of excitement quickly burst, however. By the end of 1990, researchers in Guinea-Bissau found that children who had been inoculated with the new vaccine were immune to measles but were dying at higher-than-expected rates of pneumonia, diarrhea, and parasitic diseases. But immunization against measles was supposed to bring the number of children who died from these conditions down.

Researchers in Senegal, Haiti, and other places soon reported the same problem. In June 1992, WHO temporarily halted the use of the experimental vaccine. In October 1992, the vaccine was officially scrapped.

Why were children who received the vaccine dying at higher rates than expected? "It's well known that infection with the wild-type measles virus can suppress the immune system . . ." said Dr. Diane Griffin of Johns Hopkins. "A high-dose vaccine may just mimic, in an amplified way, what happens with natural measles."[7]

One of the problems in finding a better vaccine is that there are not a lot of people involved in measles research anymore. Most of the work in developing an effective measles vaccine was done between 1954 and 1966. Within five years after the vaccine was approved in 1963 the number of cases of measles dropped 95 percent in the United States! It worked so well that less emphasis was placed on trying to find out more about measles.

Many health experts believe that the ideal vaccine will be made through genetic engineering. The vaccine would not be made with a live, weakened virus. Instead, it would contain only the parts of the virus that cause the body to produce antibodies, but not the parts that cause the immune system to be suppressed. But years of basic research on the measles virus will be needed before researchers can make an effective genetically engineered vaccine. Establishing safety may also be difficult, especially because of the experience with atypical measles when whole killed-measles vaccine was used.

One advantage of a genetically engineered vaccine is that it could be designed to include parts of a number of different disease viruses and thus, would provide protection against several diseases at the same time. The major emphasis at WHO now is on developing a multivalent vaccine (one providing protection against a number of diseases), which would be easy to administer to large groups of people.

Lives Are Being Saved

Although the battle to completely wipe out measles is still going on, much suffering has been avoided and many lives have been saved and continue to be saved because of aggressive vaccination programs. The CDC estimates that in the first twenty-five years of use, the measles vaccine has prevented nearly 75 million cases of infection in the United States. If those 75 million children had developed measles, 24,200 children might have become mentally retarded, and 7,450 would have died.[8]

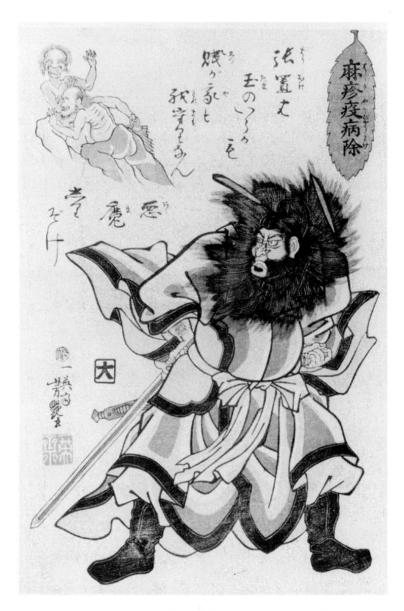

Steps are being taken all over the world to stop the spread of measles and rubella. This poster promotes a Japanese campaign against measles. Above, measles is depicted as a hairy demon.

Even though one promising vaccine did not work out, researchers worldwide are confident that, by continuing to find out more about the measles virus, they will discover better ways to outsmart it. Meanwhile, public-health efforts to increase the level of immunization may ultimately increase the herd immunity to the point where babies would not be likely to come in contact with the virus.

Most health experts are confident that through the cooperation of health officials, doctors, and the public to continue aggressive vaccination programs, measles and other childhood diseases can and will be wiped out.

Q & A

Q. What's the big fuss about measles? Isn't it just a kid's disease?

A. Measles is mainly a disease of childhood, but it can be very serious, especially when it strikes teenagers or adults. Its symptoms are like a bad case of flu with a rash, and it can lead to complications—other infections or even death. Although it is now rare in the United States, it kills more than one million children each year throughout the world.

Q. Is measles easy to catch?

A. Yes. It is one of the most contagious diseases. You can catch measles even from being in a room where an infected person was a few hours before.

Q. Can you catch measles from somebody who just got vaccinated?

A. No. Although a live virus is used for the measles vaccine, studies have shown that it is not contagious. So, you can't catch the disease (or get immunized against it) by contact with someone who has recently been vaccinated.

Q. If you have a rash, how can you tell if you have measles?

A. Many diseases produce rashes (and reactions to antibiotics such as penicillin can also produce a skin rash), so only laboratory tests can give a definite diagnosis of measles.

Q. Does the measles rash leave you with scars?

A. No, it usually disappears within a week or so. A thin layer of skin may peel afterward.

Q. What's the difference between measles and German measles?

A. Measles (rubeola) is a very serious disease and is extremely contagious. German measles (rubella) has a somewhat similar-looking rash but its symptoms are milder and it is not quite as contagious. Rubella is dangerous mainly to the children born to women who have the infection early in pregnancy.

Q. Where can I get vaccinated?

A. Family doctors, clinics, and local health departments can give immunizations. The health services of schools and colleges provide them free when there is a local measles outbreak.

Q. Why don't they give measles vaccinations to babies when they are a couple of months old?

A. Young babies get measles antibodies from their mothers before birth, and these antibodies usually last for up to fifteen months. The mother's antibodies block the baby's ability to make its own antibodies in response to measles vaccine, so the baby cannot develop lasting immunity. This causes problems in countries where measles is common, because some babies lose their mother's antibodies before it is time to get vaccinated, and then they can catch the disease. Babies born to mothers who were vaccinated rather than having a measles infection are not protected as long after birth, because vaccination produces fewer antibodies than natural measles, and the mothers have fewer antibodies to pass to their infants.

Q. If rubella is such a mild disease, except for pregnant women, why do they vaccinate boys against it, too?

A. In the United States, doctors believe that the best way to prevent rubella is to vaccinate everyone, so that the virus will become so rare that there is little chance of catching it. In some other countries, only adolescent girls are vaccinated. From the results so far, the American practice seems to be more effective in lowering the disease rates.

Q. I think I got only one measles shot. Am I protected?

A. There is about a 5 percent chance that you are not. For reliable protection it is best to have two measles vaccinations.

Measles Timeline

2500 B.C.—Probably the time when measles first became established.

900 B.C.
−500—Biblical descriptions of "plagues" may refer to measles.

A.D. **200s**—Epidemics of measles occurred in the Mediterranean region.

300s—Epidemics of measles occurred in China.

800s—Persian physician al-Rhazes described measles cases; it was thought to be a normal part of childhood.

1568—Measles carried by Spanish conquistadors helped to reduce the population of Mexico from 30 million to 3 million.

1629—English parish records list measles as a cause of death.

1657—First measles epidemic in Colonial America (in Boston).

1670—Thomas Sydenham published a medical description of measles.

1752
&1758—German physicians describe Rötheln (rubella).

1758—English physician Francis Home tried to immunize people with pus from measles sores.

1840s—The term "German measles" was first used.

1846—Danish physician P. L. Panum made detailed observations of a measles epidemic on the Faroe Islands.

1862—Louis Pasteur established that diseases were caused by germs.

1866—H. Veale first used the name "rubella."

1881—International Congress of Medicine decided rubella was a distinct disease.

1890s—Viruses were discovered and the American pediatrician Henry Koplik described characteristic Koplik spots in measles patients.

1911—Researchers produced measles in monkeys by injecting filtered material from human measles patients.

1930s—Measles viruses were first grown in tissue cultures.

1944—Australian ophthalmologist Norman McAllister Gregg proposed that rubella infection in pregnancy could lead to birth defects.

1954—John Franklin Enders isolated measles viruses.

1938—Japanese researchers showed rubella was a viral disease.

1962—Rubella virus was isolated and grown in tissue culture.

1963—Measles vaccines were available; vaccines against rubella were developed.

1969—Rubella vaccines became available.

1989—Sudden outbreaks of measles in the United States.

For More Information

Centers for Disease Control and Prevention
Public Inquiries
1600 Clifton Road, NE
Atlanta, GA 30333

Merck & Co., Inc.
One Merck Drive
P.O. Box 100
Whitehouse Station, NJ 08889

National Institute of Allergy and Infectious Disease—NIH
Bldg. 31, Room 7A-50
31 Center Drive MSC 2520
Bethesda, MD 20892

Public Health Service
Regional Office—HHS Region III
3535 Market Street
P.O. Box 13716
Philadelphia, PA 19101

World Health Organization
20 Avenue Appia
1211 Geneva 27
Switzerland

The National Vaccine Injury Compensation Program
Provides compensation (payment) for people who are
seriously injured by vaccines.
For details call (800) 338-2382.

Chapter Notes

Chapter 1

1. Max Gates, "Siena Quarantine Points to Threat of Measles Outbreak," *The Star-Ledger* (Newark, N.J.), April 9, 1989, Section 2, p. 12; Siena College news releases, February 10, 13, 14, 17, and 21, and May 9, 1989; John D'Argenio, "Siena's Sensational Season: More Than a Measles Mess," *Siena Alumni News,* Spring 1989, pp. 1, 9; Lisa Marie White, "Epidemic Leaves Mark on All Aspects of Siena Life," Ibid., pp. 1, 7; "'Green Plague?' No. 'Siena Saints,' YES!" Ibid., p. 7.

2. *Science Annual 1995* (Danbury, Conn.: Grolier, Inc., 1994), p. 366.

3. Susan Figliulo, "Measles Resurgence Puts Millions at Risk," *The Star-Ledger* (Newark, N.J.), November 5, 1989, Section 2, p. 14.

4. Devera Pine, "Comeback Diseases," *1993 Science Supplement,* p. 141.

5. Ibid.

6. *Science Annual 1995*, p. 366.

7. Ibid.

8. Michelle Healy, "Measles Epidemic Is Easing," *The Courier-News* (Bridgewater, N.J.), August 21, 1992, p. A12.

Chapter 2

1. William H. McNeill, *Plagues and People* (Garden City, N.Y.: Anchor Press/Doubleday, 1976), p. 80.

2. McNeill, p. 51; Wayne Biddle, *A Field Guide to Germs* (New York: Henry Holt & Co., 1995), p. 91.

3. Biddle, p. 92.

4. McNeill, p. 80.

5. Ibid., p. 100.

6. Ibid., p. 91.

7. James D. Cherry, "Measles," *Textbook of Pediatric Infectious Diseases*, 3rd ed., by Ralph Feigin and James D. Cherry (Philadelphia: W. B. Saunders & Co., 1992), p. 1591.

8. McNeill, pp. 117–118.

9. Ibid., p. 135.

10. Ibid., p. 117.

11. Cherry, p. 1591.

12. Ibid., p. 1592.

13. Rebecca Voelker, "Measles on the Rise," *The World Book Health & Medical Annual 1992* (Chicago: World Book, Inc., 1991), p. 30.

14. Biddle, pp. 91–93.

15. Stephen J. Ackerman, "Measles on the Rebound," *FDA Consumer*, October 1986, p. 19.

16. Frederick F. Cartwright, *Disease and History* (New York: Thomas Y. Crowell Company, 1972), p. 132.

17. Ibid., pp. 132–133.

18. McNeill, pp. 203–204.

19. Ibid., p. 210.

20. Cartwright, p. 133.

21. Ibid.; Cherry, p. 1591.

22. Cherry, p. 1592; Cartwright, pp. 134–135.

23. Cartwright, pp. 135–136; Biddle, p. 93.

24. Ibid.

25. Ibid.; Biddle, p. 93.; Ackerman, p. 20.

26. Cherry, p. 1592.

27. James D. Cherry, "Rubella," *Textbook of Pediatric Infectious Diseases*, 3rd. ed., by Ralph Feigin and James D. Cherry (Philadelphia: W. B. Saunders & Co., 1992), p. 1792.

Chapter 3

1. ". . . And Measles, Too," *FDA Consumer*, July-August 1989, p. 15.

2. Scott Minerbrook and Francesca Lunzer Kritz, "Return of a Childhood Killer," *U.S. News & World Report*, August 20, 1990, p. 64.

3. Frederick F. Cartwright, *Disease and History* (New York: Thomas Y. Crowell Company, 1972), p. 131.

4. James D. Cherry, "Measles," *Textbook of Pediatric Infectious Diseases*, 3rd ed., by Ralph Feigin and James D. Cherry (Philadelphia: W. B. Saunders & Co., 1992), p. 1595.

5. David P. Willis, "3,000 Inoculated in Measles Scare," *The Courier-News* (Bridgewater, N.J.), March 29, 1994, p. A1.

6. *Measles*, Information sheet from the New York State Department of Health.

7. Bob A. Freeman, *Burrows Textbook of Microbiology*, 22nd ed. (Philadelphia: W. B. Saunders, Co., 1985), p. 799.

8. "Measles, Mumps, and Rubella Vaccine (MMR)," Information sheet from the Centers for Disease Control, June 10, 1994.

9. Reuters, "In Finland, Exit Mumps and Measles" *The New York Times*, November 25, 1994, p. A8; Rebecca Voelker, "Measles on the Rise," *The World Book Health & Medical Annual 1992*, (Chicago: World Book, Inc., 1991), p. 32.

10. Voelker, pp. 31–32.

11. Ibid., p. 32.

12. Reuters, p. A8.

13. A. A. Milne, "Sneezles," *Now We Are Six* (New York: E. P. Dutton & Co., 1927).

14. Tina Adler, "Finding a Measles–Crohn's Disease Link," *Science News*, August 27, 1994, p. 132.

15. Lisa Belkin, "Measles, Not Yet a Thing of the Past, Reveals the Limits of an Old Vaccine," *The New York Times*, February 26, 1989, p. 22.

16. Josh Barbanel, "Many Fear Measles Tagged Along with Student," *The New York Times*, April 10, 1992, p. B6.

17. *Measles*, Information sheet from the New York State Department of Health.

18. Anne Conover Heller, "A New Rash of Measles," *Redbook*, July 1987, p. 30.

19. Freeman, p. 798; David O. White and Frank Fenner, *Medical Virology*, 3rd ed. (New York: Academic Press, Inc., 1986), p. 255.

20. Paul H. B. Shin, "N.J. Measles Cases Among Top 5 in '94," *The Courier-News* (Bridgewater, N.J.), September 5, 1995, p. A1.

21. Ibid.

22. David P. Willis, "Measles Cases Increase at Rutgers," *The Courier-News* (Bridgewater, N.J.), March 30, 1994, p A2.

Chapter 4

1. Elisabeth Rosenthal, "Rash Diagnosis," *Discover*, June 1991, p. 36.

2. Stephen J. Ackerman, "Measles on the Rebound," *FDA Consumer*, October 1986, p. 18.

3. "Your Health," *The Star-Ledger* (Newark, N.J.), April 25, 1991, p. 70; Associated Press, "Measles Risks Found Reduced by Vitamin A," *The New York Times*, July 22, 1990, p. 23.

4. Associated Press, "Measles Risks Found Reduced by Vitamin A," p. 23.

Chapter 5

1. Josh Barbanel, "Many Fear Measles Tagged Along with Student," *The New York Times*, April 10, 1992, p. B6.

2. Stephen J. Ackerman, "Measles on the Rebound," *FDA Consumer*, October 1986, p. 18.

3. Felicity T. Cutts and Lauri E. Markowitz, "Successes and Failures in Measles Control," *The Journal of Infectious Diseases*, Supplement 1, November 1994, p. S33.

4. Edna Adan Ismail, "From Surviving Smallpox to Preventing Measles," *World Health*, July 1988, p. 26.

5. Rebecca Voelker, "Measles on the Rise," *The World Book Health & Medical Annual 1992* (Chicago: World Book, Inc., 1991), p. 38.

6. Ibid., p. 29.

7. "Measles, Mumps, and Rubella Vaccine (MMR)," Information sheet from the Centers for Disease Control, June 10, 1994; *Possible Side Effects and Adverse Reactions to Measles, Mumps, and Rubella Immunization*, CDC, March 9, 1995. (On the Internet at http://www3.medaccess.com/consumer/h_child/cdcimun/measles/m1_18.htm.)

8. Voelker, p. 33.

9. "Measles, Mumps, and Rubella Vaccine (MMR)," Information sheet from the Centers for Disease Control, June 10, 1994.

10. "Measles Shots and Colds May Not Mix," *The Courier-News* (Bridgewater, N.J.), April 25, 1991, p. A3.

11. "Measles, Mumps, and Rubella Vaccine (MMR)," Information sheet from the Centers for Disease Control, June 10, 1994.

12. Irwin A. Oppenheim, "The Spotted Story About Measles After Childhood," *Current Health*, April 1987, p. 17.

13. Abram S. Benenson, ed., *Control of Communicable Diseases in Man* (Washington, D.C.: American Public Health Association, 1990), p. 274.

Chapter 6

1. James N. Baker, "Measles Busters: Chicago's Vaccine Plan," *Newsweek*, August 21, 1989, p. 22.

2. Lisa Belkin, "Measles, Not Yet a Thing of the Past, Threatens a Vast Resurgence in '89," *The New York Times*, February 26, 1989, p. 22.

3. "Eliminating Measles in the U.S.," *Medical Tribune*, July 15, 1987, p. 18.

4. Rebecca Voelker, "Measles on the Rise," *The World Book Health & Medical Annual 1992* (Chicago: World Book, Inc., 1991), p. 34.

5. Ibid., p. 36.

6. Ibid., p. 37.

7. Stephen J. Ackerman, "Measles on the Rebound," *FDA Consumer*, October 1986, p. 18.

8. Michelle Healy, "Measles Epidemic Is Easing," *The Courier-News* (Bridgewater, N.J.), August 21, 1992, p. A12.

9. Voelker, p. 37.

10. Ibid.

11. Ibid., p. 38.

12. Nancy Gagliardi, "Beware the New Measles Epidemic," *Redbook*, July 1990, p. 34.

13. "U. S. Says It's Winning the Battle Against Measles," *The New York Times*, October 29, 1993, p. A14.

14. Ibid.

15. David P. Willis, "Measles Inoculation Hits High Gear As Deadline Nears," *The Courier-News* (Bridgewater, N.J.), April 7, 1994, p. A2.

16. David P. Willis, "3,000 Inoculated in Measles Scare," *The Courier-News* (Bridgewater, N.J.), March 29, 1994, p. A1.

17. David P. Willis, "Vaccine Program Extended," *The Courier-News* (Bridgewater, N.J.), April 8, 1994, p. A2.

18. "Measles Cases Rise After Low Year," *The Courier-News* (Bridgewater, N.J.), July 8, 1995, p. A2.

19. "Measles at a Low in the Americas," *The Courier-News* (Bridgewater, N.J.), December 31, 1995, p. G1.

Chapter 7

1. David O. White and Frank Fenner, *Medical Virology*, 3rd ed. (New York: Academic Press, Inc., 1986), pp. 271, 499.

2. Peter Radetsky, *The Invisible Invaders* (Boston: Little, Brown and Company, 1991), p. 117.

3. Information sheet from the New York State Department of Health; *Rubella: More Detailed Information*, CDC, March 9, 1995. (On the Internet at http://www.medaccess.com/cdcimun/Rubella/Rub2_05.htm.)

4. *Backgrounder: Rubella*, National Institute of Allergy and Infectious Diseases, July 1991, p. 1.

5. Ibid.; Information sheet from the New York State Department of Health.

6. *Rubella*, Information sheet from the New York State Department of Health; *Rubella: Overview*, CDC, March 9, 1995. (On the Internet at http://www.medaccess.com/cdcimun/Rubella/Rub2_01.htm.)

7. White and Fenner, p. 502.

8. *Backgrounder: Rubella*, p. 2.

9. White and Fenner, p. 505.

10. Bob A. Freeman, *Burrows Textbook of Microbiology*, 22nd ed. (Philadelphia: W. B. Saunders, Co., 1985), p. 866.

11. Ibid., p. 867.

12. Abram S. Benenson, ed., *Control of Communicable Diseases in Man* (Washington, D.C.: American Public Health Association, 1990), p. 379.

13. Ibid., p. 380.

14. White and Fenner, p. 507.

Chapter 8

1. Bruce G. Gellin et al., "A Bellagio Consensus," *The Journal of Infectious Diseases*, Supplement 1, November 1994, pp. S63–S64.

2. Reuters, "In Finland, Exit Mumps and Measles," *The New York Times*, November 25, 1994, p. A8.

3. Lawrence K. Altman, "New Virus Blamed in Deaths of Australian Man and Horses," *The New York Times*, April 7, 1995, p. A20.

4. Ibid.

5. Kwai-Cheung Chan, United States General Accounting Office, *Vaccines for Children: Reexamination of Program Goals and Implementation Needed to Ensure Vaccination*, GAO/PEMD-95-22, June 1995, pp. ES-1-8.

6. Rick Weiss, "Measles Battle Loses Potent Weapon," *Science*, October 23, 1992, p. 546.

7. Ibid.

8. *The World Book Health & Medical Annual 1992* (Chicago: World Book, Inc., 1991), p. 39.

Glossary

active immunization—Producing lasting protection against a disease by injecting a substance (such as an attenuated virus) that stimulates the body's production of antibodies against the disease germ.

antibiotics—Drugs that kill bacteria or help the body to overcome them.

antibodies—Proteins produced to bind specifically to foreign chemicals (antigens), such as surface chemicals on an invading virus.

attenuated—Referring to strains of disease germs weakened by growing for a long time in animal cells or by being treated with chemicals, heat, or other factors that do not kill the germs but make them unable to cause disease.

cataract—A clouding of the eye lens that blocks vision.

congenital—Referring to a condition present at birth.

contagious—Transmissible from one person to another.

CRS—Congenital rubella syndrome: a group of birth defects associated with rubella infection of the mother during the first three months of pregnancy.

encephalitis—An inflammation of the brain.

endemic disease—A disease that is usually present in the population.

epidemic—An infectious disease that spreads over a wide area in a limited span of time.

gamma globulin—A blood product consisting of one type of antibodies from someone who has been exposed to disease-causing germs.

German measles—Another name for rubella.

herd immunity—A general resistance of the population to a disease that exists when there are not enough susceptible individuals to keep the chain of infection going.

immune globulin—A blood product consisting of antibodies from someone who has been exposed to specific disease-causing germs.

immune system—Various body defenses against invading microbes, including white blood cells and interferon.

immunoglobulin (IG)—A blood fraction containing antibodies against disease microbes.

incubation period—The time between infection and appearance of symptoms.

inflammation—Swelling, pain, heat, and redness in the tissues around a site of infection.

interferon—A protein released by virus-infected cells that protects other cells from infection.

killed-virus vaccine—A vaccine made from viruses that have been killed.

Koplik spots—An early sign of measles: small blue-white spots surrounded by red rings, which appear on the inside of the cheeks.

live-virus vaccine—A vaccine made from live viruses, capable of infecting humans but not of causing disease.

MMR—Measles-mumps-rubella vaccine.

morbilli—Another name for measles.

morbilliform rash—A typical measles rash consisting of flat reddish-brown lesions, which join together to form large blotches and leave a brownish stain when the rash fades.

Morbillivirus—The genus to which measles virus belongs.

MR—Measles-rubella vaccine.

nucleic acid—A type of biochemical that contains hereditary instructions.

paramyxovirus—A family of viruses including those that cause measles and mumps (but not rubella).

passive immunization—Providing temporary protection against a disease by injecting antibodies against the disease germ, taken from the blood of people who are immune to it.

pneumonia—A serious illness with sharp chest pain, severe cough, and very high fever, due to infection of lung tissue by viruses or bacteria.

polyvalent vaccine—A combined vaccine that provides protection against several diseases, such as MMR.

Reye's syndrome—A rare but serious illness associated with taking aspirin during a viral infection.

rubelliform rash—A typical rubella rash consisting of pink, pin-sized lesions that remain separated and disappear relatively quickly.

rubivirus—The genus to which the rubella virus belongs.

seizure—A condition in which a person may stare, unaware of the surroundings, and jerk or go into convulsions.

togaviridae—The virus family that includes the rubella virus.

vaccination—Administration (usually by injection or orally) of a preparation of microbes or their products to stimulate protective immunity against disease.

wild-type virus—The form of a virus that circulates naturally in the population.

Further Reading

Books

Biddle, Wayne. *A Field Guide to Germs*. New York: Henry Holt & Co., 1995.

Cartwright, Frederick F. *Disease and History*. New York: Thomas Y. Crowell Company, 1972.

Cherry, James D. "Measles," *Textbook of Pediatric Infectious Diseases*, 3rd ed., by Ralph Feigin and James D. Cherry. Philadelphia: W. B. Saunders & Co., 1992.

McNeill, William H. *Plagues and People*. Garden City, NY: Anchor Press/Doubleday, 1976.

Metos, Thomas H. *Communicable Diseases*. New York: Franklin Watts, 1987.

Radetsky, Peter. *The Invisible Invaders*. Boston: Little, Brown and Company, 1991.

Van Dijk, Jan. *Persons Handicapped by Rubella: Victors and Victims—A Follow-Up Study*. Amsterdam: Swets & Zeitlinger, 1991.

Articles:

Abella, Mary. "Measles Menace." *Better Homes and Gardens*, November 1990, p. 51.

Ackerman, Stephen J. "Measles on the Rebound." *FDA Consumer*, October 1986, pp. 18–21.

Altman, Lawrence K. "New Virus Blamed in Deaths of Australian Man and Horses." *The New York Times*, April 7, 1995, p. A20.

―――. "Scientists, Hoping to End Measles, Find a Surprisingly Resilient Foe." *The New York Times*, March 28, 1989, p. C3.

Brody, Jane E. "Resurgence of Measles Across the Nation Prompts New Recommendations on Vaccinations." *The New York Times*, January 11, 1990, p. B10.

Gagliardi, Nancy. "Beware the New Measles Epidemic." *Redbook*, July 1990, pp. 34–36.

Heller, Anne Conover. "A New Rash of Measles." *Redbook*, July 1987, p. 30.

"Measles Control—Resetting the Agenda: A Report of the Children's Vaccine Initiative Ad Hoc Committee on an Investment Strategy for Measles Control." *The Journal of Infectious Diseases*, November 1994, Supplement 1.

Minerbrook, Scott and Francesca Lunzor Kritz. "Return of a Childhood Killer." *U.S. News & World Report*, August 20, 1990, pp. 63–64.

Oppenheim, Irwin A. "The Spotted Story About Measles After Childhood." *Current Health 2*, April 1987, pp. 16–17.

Rosenthal, Elisabeth. "Rash Diagnosis." *Discover*, June 1991, pp. 36–39.

―――. "Resurgent Measles Much Worse Than a Nuisance." *The New York Times*, April 24, 1991, pp. A1, A18.

Rossen, Anne E. "Comeback Diseases." *Current Health*, January 1991, pp. 26–27.

Stevens, William K. "Despite Vaccine, Perilous Measles Won't Go Away." *The New York Times*, March 14, 1989, pp. C1, C6.

Voelker, Rebecca. "Measles on the Rise." *World Book Health & Medical Annual 1992*, pp. 28–39.

Weiss, Rick. "Measles Battle Loses Potent Weapon." *Science*, October 1992, pp. 546–547.

Pamphlets

The World Health Organization offers a number of free pamphlets, reprints, charts, and slides on measles and the worldwide efforts to control it.

Internet Sources

Helpful text and interesting pictures can be found at the following sites:

http://KidsHealth.org/parent/healthy [Childhood Infections]

http://medhlp.netusa.net [Med Help International]

http://www.cdc.gov [Centers for Disease Control and Prevention]

http://www.merck.com [Merck & Co.]

http://www.nlm.nih.gov [National Library of Medicine]

http://www.who.ch [World Health Organization]

Index